Keeping a healthy heart,
with important information from:

William Castelli, M.D., Director of the Framingham Heart Study, on cholesterol and heart disease.

Earl Benditt, M.D., of the University of Washington, on tumors in the heart.

Michael DeBakey, M.D., Heart surgeon, Methodist Hospital, Houston, Texas, on preventing heart disease.

Vital facts on preventing cancer
with the perspectives of:

John Bailar, M.D., Ph.D., former Editor-in-Chief of the *Journal of the National Cancer Institute*, on redirecting the "War on Cancer."

Oliver Alabaster, M.D., of the George Washington University Medical Center, on how food choices prevent cancer.

Peter Greenwald, M.D., of the National Cancer Institute, on how vitamins in foods can prevent cancer.

Denis Burkitt, M.D., leading authority on fiber, on how fiber protects against cancer of the colon and breast.

The latest on controlling your weight,
with vital information from:

William Connor, M.D., of the University of Oregon, on how food selections help control weight.

C. Wayne Callaway, M.D., formerly of the Mayo Clinic and the George Washington University Medical Center, on how timing factors affect weight.

Contaminants of all kinds in our foods,
and what to do about them, with:

Carol Tucker Foreman, former Assistant Secretary of Agriculture, on what you didn't know was in your grocery bag.

Mitchell Cohen, M.D., of the Centers for Disease Control, on how bacteria in foods can cause illness.

D0047135

Surprising new ways
to prevent a broad range of illnesses, with:

Denis Burkitt, M.D., on how food choices lead to common conditions, from cancer to varicose veins.

John McDougall, M.D., physician, medical lecturer, and author, on food choices in osteoporosis, kidney disease, and other common problems.

Monroe Rosenthal, M.D., Medical Director of the Pritikin Program, on the role of foods in diabetes and other conditions.

How what you eat affects
your mood and mental functioning, with:

Richard Wurtman, M.D., of the Massachusetts Institute of Technology, on how foods affect brain chemistry.

C. Keith Conners, Ph.D., of Children's Hospital in Washington, D.C., on how foods affect the child's mind and behavior.

Insights on our natural diet, from:

Jane Goodall, Ph.D., renowned primatologist, on the natural diet of primates.

Richard Leakey, Ph.D., paleoanthropologist, on the evolution of the human diet.

Surprising findings from Asia, with:

T. Colin Campbell, Ph.D., of Cornell University, the head of the China Diet and Health Study, on what Asian diets can tell us about our own.

Anthony Sattilaro, M.D., former President of Methodist Hospital, Philadelphia, on foods as a treatment for cancer.

THE
POWER
OF YOUR
PLATE

A Plan for Better Living
Eating well for better health—
20 experts tell you how!

By Neal D. Barnard, M.D.
Author of *Food For Life*

Book Publishing Company ◆ Summertown, Tennessee

Cover design by Doug Hall

Barnard, Neal., 1953-
    The power of your plate : a plan for better living / by Neal
D. Barnard, author of Food for life.
        p. cm.
    Previously published: 1990
    Includes bibliographical references and index.
    ISBN 1-57067-003-X
    1. Nutrition. 2. Nutritionally induced diseases. I. Title.
QP141,B263
612.3--dc20   94-43222
                                                  CIP

Also by Dr. Barnard:
    A Physician's Slimming Guide Summertown, TN: Book Publishing
        Company, 1992
    Live Longer, Live Better Cassette. Summertown, TN: Book Pub-
        lishing Company, 1992
    Food for Life New York, NY: Harmony Books, 1993

Notice to Readers

This book provides detailed information on how food choices improve health. It does not take the place of individualized medical care. If you have any medical condition, are taking medication, or are over forty, please see your doctor before changing your diet or increasing your physical activity. Changes in diet and exercise sometimes necessitate a change in medications or in other aspects of medical care.

Vegetarian diets are very powerful and healthful. Assuring an appropriate intake of vitamin B-12 does require a little planning, however, so please consult the simple guidelines on page 197. This is important for everyone, but particularly for children and pregnant or nursing women.

The animal-based diet that most Westerners currently follow is risky. If you are on such a diet and, for whatever reason, you decide to stay on it, please see your physician regularly, continue to read about the value of changing your diet, and please encourage others not to follow your example.

Similarly, diets based on poultry or fish are extremely weak and are not recommended. They do not provide the cholesterol-lowering, weight-reducing, or cancer-preventive effects that come from a plant-based diet, and they do not reverse heart disease in most patients.

If you would like additional information about nutrition and health issues, let me encourage you to subscribe to *Good Medicine*, a quarterly magazine published by the Physicians Committee for Responsible Medicine. It is available for an annual subscription price of $20 from PCRM, Box 6322, Washington, D.C. 20015. I can be reached at the same address, and would very much like to hear how you are doing with your new program for health. Good luck!

Neal D. Barnard, M.D.

Table of Contents

Introduction

Healthy eating is a gold mine. With the right food selections, you can lose weight permanently, without restrictive diets. You can prevent heart attacks and even reverse existing heart disease. Through a combined approach of life-style changes, as much as eighty percent of cancer can be prevented. Millions of cases of what passes for the "flu" actually came into our homes in our groceries. We can prevent those as well. We can use foods to get a good night's sleep without sleeping pills, and can plan a morning meal that will help us feel alert through the day.

We will look at the best and latest information on healthy eating from leading authorities. These experts usually write for other scientists and doctors, rather than for the lay public. But they have found the very best ways to control weight permanently, to lower cholesterol dramatically, to prevent cancer, and to do many other things through simple and straightforward food choices. You should know about it.

Many of the things I discovered in preparing this book surprised me too. As a doctor, I knew about the importance of nutrition, but, like most physicians, I began my career without taking the time to look at the real state of the art in nutrition research. Years ago, when the University Hospital swallowed me along with the other frightened medical students, we had too much on our minds to think about healthy eating. Our neckties were awkwardly knotted under our collars. Our white jackets were baggy and too short. We were terrified of drowning in the long hours of demanding, detailed work. Nutrition, preventive medicine, and health in general never figured in our minds. With junk food stuffed in our pockets and plenty of black coffee and cigarettes, we were determined only to survive.

Near the end of my medical training, however, I found that there is a wealth of information which is well-known to researchers, but is largely unknown to lay readers. For example:

* **The best plans for weight loss** are based, not on how much you eat, but on what you eat and when. Weight control can be maintained while actually eating more calories than are consumed by most overweight people.

* **Specific steps** can increase your ability to burn off calories and trim your waistline more effectively than "diets" ever could.

* **Eighty percent of cancer** can potentially be prevented by steps we can take ourselves.

* **Our moods and alertness** are distinctly altered by the balance of nutrients in our diet. Certain foods are used as building blocks for chemicals in the brain.

* **New evidence shows that heart disease** can not only be prevented; even long-standing disease can be reversed.

* **Chicken and fish are not health foods.** They are overly high in protein and chemical and bacterial contaminants, and they are not as low in fat and cholesterol as you might think.

* **Protein can be damaging** to both kidney function and calcium metabolism when ingested in more than moderate amounts.

* **Infectious agents and chemical residues** are common in many foods and cause millions of cases of illness each year, including "flu"-like syndromes and serious birth defects.

In this book, I have let leaders in research tell of their findings themselves:

C. Wayne Callaway, M.D., of the George Washington University, and *William Connor, M.D.*, of the University of Oregon, detail the new weight control strategies.

Oliver Alabaster, M.D., the Director of the Institute for Disease Prevention at the George Washington University Medical Center, *John Bailar, M.D., Ph.D.*, former Editor-in-Chief of the Journal of the National Cancer Institute, *Peter Greenwald, M.D.*, Director of Cancer Prevention and Control of the National Cancer Institute, and *Denis Burkitt, M.D.*, the renowned surgeon and pioneering researcher on the value of fiber, tell of the War on Cancer and the breakthrough dietary approach to cancer prevention.

Heart surgeon *Michael DeBakey, M.D.*, *William Castelli, M.D.*, of the Framingham Heart Study, and *Earl Benditt, M.D.*, of the University of Washington, tell of the new approaches to cholesterol and heart disease.

Denis Burkitt, M.D., whose expertise covers not only cancer research but research into other common illnesses as well, *John McDougall, M.D.*, a leading author and lecturer on nutrition, and *Monroe Rosenthal, M.D.*, of the Pritikin Program, describe the new approaches to a variety of common illnesses from constipation to varicose veins to osteoporosis and impotence.

Mitchell Cohen, M.D., of the Centers for Disease Control, and *Carol Tucker Foreman*, the former Assistant Secretary of Agriculture, tell of the uninvited guests that lurk in foods.

Richard Wurtman, M.D., of the Massachusetts Institute of Technology, and *C. Keith Conners, Ph.D.*, of Children's Hospital in Washington, D.C., detail the effects of foods on the mental functioning of children and adults.

Leading primate expert *Jane Goodall* and paleoanthropologist *Richard E. Leakey* give fascinating insights into the evolution of the human diet.

T. Colin Campbell, Ph.D. and *Anthony Sattilaro, M.D.*, show how traditional Asian diets give a fresh perspective on our own.

In engaging interviews, they tell of their unique perspectives on the power of foods. Each of them has broken new ground. They might not agree totally with each other or with me at times, but each offers an essential piece of the puzzle. From their comments and from the medical literature I have drawn simple but far-reaching recommendations for an optimal menu. In a final section, we will look in depth at how to change long-standing habits. The human animal keeps a tenacious grip on old food habits. By taking human psychology into account, we can begin a new and healthful menu.

I owe a debt of gratitude to the individuals whose words are printed in this volume. They shared not only their expertise and unique ideas, but also a substantial amount of time and many helpful suggestions. Special thanks also go to Loretta and Bob Hirsh for their encouragement and innumerable leads to new perspectives.

Chapter 1

Cholesterol, Food, and Your Heart

Every day, 4,000 Americans have a heart attack. Those who survive often suffer another heart attack later. But this does not have to occur. To a great extent, we can now control the risk of heart attacks. And we can even reverse existing heart disease.

The key is to control what are called "risk factors." Studies show that the likelihood of heart attacks increases when high cholesterol levels, smoking, sedentary life-style, or high blood pressure are present. When these specific risk factors are under good control, the risk of heart trouble plummets.

Other factors also contribute to risk: diabetes, obesity, family history of heart disease, stress, and the "Type A" personality characterized by a need to excel, bossiness, time urgency, and impatience. Some of these cannot be changed. But by simply controlling our diet, smoking, and exercise habits, we have a tremendous amount of control over the risk of heart disease.

What is Atherosclerosis?

Before I entered medical school, I worked as a pathology assistant in a hospital morgue. It was in that desolate museum of medical history that I first saw heart disease. The pathologist would explain the autopsy findings to me as he did his examination.

"This is garden-variety atherosclerosis," he said as his scissors went crunch, crunch, crunch, through the coronary arteries, one of which he sliced open. "This is what cholesterol does. We'll see this again in the carotid arteries." And sure enough, the carotids, the main arteries to the brain, were nearly closed off by swollen areas in the artery wall, called plaques. As we finished and I carefully replaced the section of ribs that had been removed to do the examination, I thought about how almost all the autopsies showed some of this deadly process, even for fairly young people.

Once, after a particularly long procedure, I raced to the hospital cafeteria for lunch. As I removed the lid from the plate, an overturned chicken breast with ribs looking precisely like the chest we had just closed, greeted me with a smell of dead tissue. The connection between diet and death could not have been more graphic.

Atherosclerosis is the all-too-common form of heart disease in which plaques of cholesterol and other substances form in the artery walls. It is one kind of *arteriosclerosis*, a general term meaning thickening and loss of elasticity of arteries.

Plaques form very much like small tumors. The process is gradual: As fats and cholesterol deposit in the walls of our arteries, the muscle cells which normally wrap around arteries, giving them strength like steel bands in a tire, start to overgrow. The muscle cells begin to multiply out of control. They form what are essentially tumors inside the artery. These are the plaques—cholesterol, fat, muscle cells, and other debris. They look like bumps on the inside wall of the artery.

The coronary arteries bring oxygen to the heart muscle itself. (They are called coronary arteries because they form a ring around the heart, rather like a crown.) As plaques gradually form, the passageway for blood becomes clogged. Less blood flow means less oxygen for the heart muscle. The heart, then, tires easily during exercise or excitement. Chest pain (angina) occurs. When the blood supply is completely blocked, a part of the heart muscle dies. This is a heart attack (myocardial infarction).

This process also occurs in the arteries to the brain and can result in a stroke, the death of a portion of the brain. When atherosclerosis compromises the arteries to the legs, the result may be severe leg pains during walking, called claudication. The process even affects the arteries to the genital area, causing impotence in men.

Atherosclerosis is not caused by old age. In affluent countries like the U.S., the early changes of atherosclerosis start in childhood. When battlefield casualties were examined in the Korean and Vietnam wars, American soldiers had significant atherosclerosis at only 18 or 20 years of age. Their Asian counterparts had much healthier arteries. At the risk of getting ahead of ourselves, you can guess what caused the difference: the Americans had been eating lots of meat and dairy products all their lives, while the Asians had been eating mainly rice and vegetables. The point is this: The reason older people are more likely to have heart problems is mainly because they have been eating badly (or smoking) longer than young people have. But, in general, people who do not do these things never need to develop atherosclerosis no matter how old they are. Old age, in and of itself, is not the cause.

Young Man, Troubled Heart

A 49-year-old man began to experience angina. Initially, the chest pain only occurred when he really overexerted himself. But things progressed very rapidly to the point where, if he walked even one block, the pain in his chest forced him to stop.

His doctor ran several tests and tried a number of medications, which helped a little. But by no means did they return him to normal. Even at the best of times, he couldn't go beyond a block. He was on a tether that was getting shorter and shorter.

Desperate, and with no more than the half-hearted blessing of his regular doctor, he joined a program of diet, exercise, and nutritional education under the guidance of a new doctor. He learned that atherosclerosis was related to diet and other factors he could control. He began with mild exercise and a meal plan that he felt was really revolutionary for him. His family changed its diet in the same way, eliminating meats and increasing vegetable foods. His health and vitality turned the corner.

Soon, he was not only walking again, he was running. When he was jogging three miles a day, he went back to show his previous doctor, who now refers many patients to the program that worked so well. His dim future of a few months before was rejuvenated into a new life. The key elements were, first of all, a major change in diet, and second, regular exercise.

A New Cholesterol Goal

Many studies have shown the connection between cholesterol and heart troubles. Beginning in 1949, the population of Framingham, Massachusetts, has been monitored to see what affects the rate of heart problems. Under the direction of William Castelli, M.D., the study is looking at an entire generation and now, its children.[1]

The Framingham study showed how common heart attacks really are. Healthy men and women were rapidly being picked off by heart disease. In the first 14 years of the study, heart attacks hit one out of every eight men who had been in their early forties at the beginning of the study. Heart attacks felled one out of four who were in their late fifties at the beginning of the study. "When our friends saw those rates," Castelli said, "they all said, 'If I were you I'd get out of Framingham.'"

Not that that would help. Lowering the level of cholesterol in your blood stream, on the other hand, can make all the difference in the world. Castelli found that there is a cholesterol level below which heart attacks essentially do not occur. "We think there is a threshold in cholesterol, and that it's 150," says Castelli. "We've never had a heart attack in Framingham in thirty-five years in anyone who had a cholesterol under 150. Three-quarters of the people who live on the face of this earth never have a heart attack. Their cholesterols are all around 150. They live in Asia, Africa, South America, outside the big cities. All they need to do to get this disease today is to make a lot of money and move to Rio or Buenos Aires or Cape Town or Singapore or Hong Kong or, lately, to Tokyo, and they can get this disease."

With the move to the big city comes an increase in meat consumption. We need to do just the reverse. If we adopt a healthier diet, we can cut our cholesterol levels and our risk of a heart attack.

Cholesterol levels are measured in milligrams (mg) of cholesterol per deciliter (dl) of blood serum. The ideal level, then, is below 150 mg/dl. At that point, a heart attack is very unlikely. Unfortunately, Americans have a long way to go. The average cholesterol in America is about 205. This is frighteningly close to 244 which is the average for heart attack victims. Some doctors still consider a cholesterol level of 244 entirely normal.

> *"We've never had a heart attack in Framingham in thirty-five years in anyone who had a cholesterol under 150. Three-quarters of the people who live on the face of this earth never have a heart attack."*
>
> **Dr. William Castelli**

A reading of 150 is lower than the level generally quoted by doctors, who often use 200 as the recommended level. The difference is this: In general, the lower one's cholesterol level, the better, until you get to about 150. Below that point, there is no great benefit to a lower cholesterol (although there is no harm in a lower level). It certainly would be a tremendous improvement if the American population had an average cholesterol below 180 or even 200. But even at those levels, some people will still develop heart disease. It is useful to remember 150 as the number below which heart disease is nearly impossible.

There is more good news. Lowering cholesterol has a two-for-one benefit. For every one percent that you reduce your cholesterol, you will have a two percent reduction in heart disease risk.[2] For example, lowering your cholesterol from 300 mg/dl to 200 mg/dl, a reduction of one-third, will give you a two-thirds reduction in risk. For some people the benefits are even greater.

Different Types of Cholesterol: HDL and LDL

Cholesterol travels in the blood in special "packages" called lipoproteins. Low density lipoproteins (LDL) and very low density lipoproteins (VLDL) are made of fat, protein, and cholesterol. LDL is known as the "bad cholesterol." The more LDL, the greater your risk of heart disease.

Cholesterol Levels

244: Average Heart Attack Victim

205: Average American

200 or less: Recommended Level by Federal Government

150 or less: Almost No Risk of Heart Disease

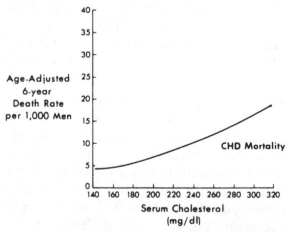

Martin MJ et al. Serum cholesterol, blood pressure, and mortality. *Lancet* 1986;2:933-36. c by The Lancet Ltd. 1986.

—Age-adjusted 6-year CHD and total mortality per 1000 men screened for MRFIT according to serum cholesterol.

High density lipoproteins (HDL) are a very different cholesterol package. Some call HDL the "good cholesterol," because it acts like little dump trucks carrying cholesterol away. HDL lowers the risk of heart disease. In general, the higher your HDL, the better. Vigorous exercise increases HDL. Modest alcohol consumption raises HDL. (While this is a comfort to those who think of alcohol as a healthy part of the grain group of foods, more than one or two drinks per day takes away any possible advantage of alcohol consumption.) Smoking and obesity appear to lower HDL.

Doctors sometimes use the ratio of total cholesterol to HDL as a predictor of heart disease risk that is better than total cholesterol alone. The ratio of total cholesterol to HDL should be below 3.5 to 1. Most Americans, unfortunately, are not yet at that safe level. The average American male's ratio is 5.1 to 1. For Boston Marathon runners the ratio averages 3.5 to 1. Vegetarians, especially those who avoid eggs and dairy products, do the best, averaging about 2.9 to 1.[1] If your total cholesterol is below 150, however, your risk is so low that your HDL level makes little difference.

Taking Control of Cholesterol

We have a tremendous degree of control over our cholesterol levels. High cholesterols do not come from the air. They come from our plates. There are, in fact, several things we put on our plates that affect our cholesterol levels. The first, of course, is cholesterol itself.

Cholesterol is found in all foods that come from animals: meat, poultry, fish, eggs, milk, cheese, yogurt, and every other meat and dairy product.

Animals, including the human animal, manufacture cholesterol in their livers for use as a building block for sex hormones, cell membranes, and digestive secretions. While the body uses cholesterol for these purposes, it makes plenty of cholesterol for all its needs. We do not need to add any more through our foods. When we do, the result is that cholesterol is left where it does not belong—in plaques in our arteries. The more cholesterol we consume, the higher our cholesterol levels go.

As a rule of thumb, for every 100 mg of cholesterol you ingest in foods on a daily basis, your cholesterol level will rise about five points. Eggs are a good example. An average egg yolk contains more than 200 mg of cholesterol. Over the long run, an egg every day can raise your cholesterol level by as much as ten points. Eggs are certainly among the worst offenders. There are others as well, as we will see. Let's look at what we can do if we eliminate cholesterol-containing foods:

A typical American might eat about 400 mg of cholesterol each day in foods. If animal products are eliminated from the diet the cholesterol level will drop significantly—about five points for every 100 mg of cholesterol eliminated from the diet. If all cholesterol is eliminated from the diet, the serum cholesterol can drop about 20 points.

$$400 \text{ mg of cholesterol eliminated} \times \frac{5 \text{ mg/dl drop}}{100 \text{ mg}} = 20 \text{ points}$$

To take this example a step further, let's imagine that a person's cholesterol drops 20 points from the American average of 205 to 185. That change alone, about 10 percent, is good for about a 20 percent reduction in risk of heart disease (the two-for-one benefit).

The effects will actually be much more profound, because, as we will see shortly, the reduction in saturated fat that goes along with cutting out cholesterol-laden foods reduces cholesterol levels even more. So cutting these foods out of the diet is a powerful step. It is easy to know where cholesterol is. Cholesterol is found in all animal products. No foods from plants contain cholesterol.

If you had thought that chicken was a health food, I am sorry to tell you that chicken contains the same amount of cholesterol as beef: 25 mg per ounce.[3] Chicken can be slightly lower in fat, but cholesterol is primarily in the lean portion of meats. So while trimming the fat will help, it will not eliminate cholesterol from meats. As we will see, there are much better answers to the cholesterol problem.

Saturated Fats

Saturated fats are cholesterol-makers. They turn on the cholesterol-producing machinery in your liver. Don't get nervous about these chemical terms. *Saturated* simply means that the fat molecule is covered with hydrogen atoms. A molecule of saturated fat is like a bus with every seat filled. There is no room for another hydrogen atom. The hydrogen atoms generally add on in pairs. If several pairs of "seats" are empty, the fat molecule is called *polyunsaturated*. If just one pair of "seats" is empty, the fat molecule is called *monounsaturated*.

An easy way to identify saturated fats is to note that they are usually solid at room temperature. Beef fat, chicken fat, and most other animal fats are largely saturated. Meats often have fat not only on the outer edge, but also marbled throughout the lean. The worst offenders are processed meats: hot dogs, salami, sausage, bologna, etc. Commercial hamburgers are in much the same category. Castelli says, "When you see the Golden Arches, you're probably on the road to the pearly gates." Even "lean" meats and poultry contain significant amounts of saturated fat (in addition to cholesterol itself).

Vegetable oils are very different. They are high in polyunsaturates or monounsaturates and generally do not raise cholesterol levels, at least not very much. Corn oil, peanut oil, safflower oil, olive oil, and other vegetable oils are in this category.

Tropical oils are exceptions; palm oil, palm kernel oil, and coconut oil are high in saturated fat. They should be avoided. To remember them, picture a palm tree with its coconuts. Read the labels on baked goods. You'll often find tropical oils in commercial products, because they resist oxidation and prolong the shelf-life of products.

Vegetable oils can be chemically changed to saturated fats by a process called hydrogenation. Hydrogenated vegetable oils, then, are solid at room temperature, so they can be used in products such as margarine and maintain a longer shelf-life. But in the process, they are turned into a fat that will raise serum cholesterol.

Doctors have tried to get patients to reduce animal fats and increase use of vegetable oils. This is good advice as far as it goes. But the best advice is to greatly reduce *all* fats and oils, whether they are saturated, polyunsaturated, or monounsaturated. While animal fats are obviously on the bad list, vegetable oils should be minimized as well. The reason is that all fats and oils—animal, vegetable, whatever—are mixtures containing at least some saturated fat, even though animal fats have much more than vegetable oils do. Also, they all seem to increase cancer risk, particularly for cancers of the breast, colon, and prostate, as we will see in detail later in this book.[4]

The bottom line is that saturated fats are the worst cholesterol-makers. They are found in meats, poultry, dairy products, and some fried and baked goods. The key to dealing with heart disease is to learn to incorporate foods from plants—grains, legumes, vegetables, and fruits—in our daily menu and to phase out animal products. The farther we move in that direction the better. A vegetarian diet is the best. More modest changes lead to modest results.

Fiber

Dietary fiber does many good things for health, including lowering cholesterol levels. It is not entirely clear why a high-fiber diet lowers cholesterol levels in the blood. Partly it is because high-fiber foods contain little fat and no cholesterol and displace some of the fatty foods from the diet.

However, some researchers have suggested that fiber, particularly soluble fiber such as is found in oatmeal or beans, can actually work like a medication to bring down cholesterol levels.[5] One theory is that fiber traps cholesterol in the digestive tract. The liver converts cholesterol into digestive secretions. They travel from the liver, down the bile ducts, and into the intestine. There, fiber soaks them up and prevents them from being reabsorbed and converted back into cholesterol. Another theory suggests that the fermentation of fiber in the colon releases short-chain fatty acids which cause the liver to reduce production of cholesterol.

In any case, you can get a tremendous benefit from changing your daily menu. You already wanted to get rid of the eggs and bacon, because they contain loads of fat and cholesterol. And when you replace them with hot cereals, low-fat bran muffins, or whole grain toast, you get a cholesterol-free meal that is also rich in fiber. Foods from animal sources—meat and dairy products—which always contain cholesterol and never contain fiber—are replaced with foods from the plant kingdom, which never contain cholesterol and are often rich in fiber.

Medication

For people with extremely high cholesterol levels, medications can be helpful in reducing them. *Cholestyramine*, for example, has been shown to lower cholesterol levels and to lead to a corresponding decrease in risk of heart attacks. It is a gritty substance that must be taken several times a day. *Colestipol* is a similarly effective cholesterol-binding agent. *Niacin*, a B vitamin, has been used to lower cholesterol. It has the disadvantages of causing a hot, flushing sensation in some people and raising blood levels of uric acid, which is responsible for gout. *Lovastatin* is effective in lowering cholesterol, but is quite expensive and, in some cases, may cause liver damage. None of these medications takes the place of food selection as the first line of defense against high cholesterol. They should be used *with* a low-fat, vegetarian diet, not *instead* of it.

Cholesterol can be raised by birth control pills and other medications. Ironically, some drugs used to treat high blood pressure may actually raise serum cholesterol. Thiazide diuretics, which are among the most commonly prescribed drugs for hypertension, have this effect, although it may be short lived.[6,7,8]

Heredity

For the vast majority of people, heredity is not an important factor in the tendency toward heart disease. A small fraction of the population, however, does have an inherited tendency toward high cholesterol levels. For some, fats in the blood stream are phenomenally elevated.

Those with a hereditary problem require careful attention to their cholesterol levels. They should shift to a low-fat, vegetarian menu. For some, medications will be necessary. But it must be emphasized: The majority of the American public has elevated cholesterol levels, and they are almost entirely due to our choice of food rather than our "choice of parents." Even in those cases where heart disease runs in families, it is often due, not to heredity, but to eating habits that persist across generations.

The Fish Oil Controversy

A recent fad was to consume fish oils in hopes of reducing cholesterol levels. It turns out that, although fish oils can lower triglyceride levels somewhat, they do not lower cholesterol levels. In fact, like all animal products, fish contain cholesterol. Species vary, but some, particularly mobile shellfish such as shrimp, lobster, or crayfish, are extremely high in cholesterol. Ounce for ounce, shrimp have 70 percent more cholesterol than beef.[3]

In addition, fish fats, like all fats, are mixtures containing a significant amount of saturated fat. The saturated portion is usually about 15 to 30 percent of the total fat content. This is lower than for beef or chicken, but still totally out of the league of grains, beans, vegetables, and fruits. Take Chinook salmon, for example. If you check its fat content, it turns out to be no less than 52 percent fat, about a quarter of which is nothing but artery-clogging saturated fat. This is part of the reason that programs seeking to reverse heart disease leave fish out of the diet.

Many research studies have shown that fish oils impair the body's immune responses to bacteria and viruses.[9,10] Of course, the most notorious problem with fish is chemical contamination, which is discussed in detail in Chapter Five. There is no advantage to including fish in the diet, and plenty of reasons to steer clear of it.

Reversing Heart Disease

If we have advanced atherosclerosis, can we become healthy again? Happily, the answer is "Yes."

For most of us, plaques form gradually over many years. They begin to clog the arteries that carry oxygen to the heart muscle. They form in the arteries to the brain or to other parts of the body. They eventually lead to serious disability, then death. But, according to Castelli, diet can reverse this process.

"I worked in the 1950s for a pathologist in Belgium," Castelli said. "Every time he did an autopsy he would say, 'They're coming back.'

"We'd say, 'What are coming back?'

"He'd say, 'The plaques are coming back.'

"'Where did they go?'

"He'd say, 'I don't know where they went, but they disappeared.'

"'When did they disappear?'

"'1942.'

"Two years after the German occupation, they disappeared from the arteries of Belgians. Before the war they were there on about three-fourths of the people who died. They disappeared from '42 to '50, not just in Belgium, but in Holland, Poland, Norway, and northern France. The Germans went into all these countries. They backed up trucks to the farms and took all the meat and livestock back to Germany with the able-bodied men to take care of them.

"And so, they went on a vegetarian diet, not because they had read Adele Davis or Nathan Pritikin—there just wasn't any meat to eat, and the lesions disappeared. And of course, now they are back. They're there now on three-fourths of the people who die."

We can get rid of the disease. Evidence shows that plaques can gradually dissolve. Atherosclerosis appears to be reversible. "It will go away," Castelli said. "Get your total cholesterol down to 150, and keep it there for five years. I don't care how you do it. Diet would be the best way, but if you have to use drugs you can still do it. You will reverse your lesions."

A number of studies have suggested that even established plaques can be diminished. Dean Ornish, M.D., is the author of *Dr. Dean Ornish's Program for Reversing Heart Disease* (Random House, 1990). Ornish and his colleagues in San Francisco have shown that a program of exercise, elimination of smoking, stress reduction, and a low-fat, vegetarian diet can yield signs of reversal within one year in 82 percent of patients. It happens gradually. But it will generally not happen unless one's life-style is comprehensively changed. The typical American Heart Association diet, composed of poultry, fish, and "lean meats," is too weak to reverse heart disease for most people. A vegetarian diet is much more powerful.

Dietary Factors in Hypertension

High blood pressure is an important contributor to heart disease. But blood pressure can often be reduced by food choices.

For everyone with high blood pressure, reduction in salt intake is a first step that your doctor will recommend. Leaving the salt shaker on the shelf helps reduce blood pressure.

A low-fat, high-carbohydrate diet, particularly a vegetarian diet, is also very helpful in lowering blood pressure. Researchers in Australia noted that vegetarians tend to have relatively low blood pressure. So they conducted a series of experiments in which people were put on a vegetarian diet for six weeks. They found a distinct drop in blood pressure. After resuming their normal diet, blood pressures went back up. The effect was shown both in normal subjects and in those with mild hypertension."[11]

It is not clear exactly why these dietary factors lower blood pressure. Researchers suggest that high-fat diets increase the tendency of blood cells to clump together and make the blood thicker (more viscous). Vegetarians tend to have significantly lower blood viscosity than meat-eaters.[12]

An interesting detail is that licorice ingestion, over the long-term, can elevate blood pressure. Certain chemicals in licorice affect the levels of sodium, potassium, and other chemicals in the blood, leading to hypertension.[13]

Weight reduction also helps lower blood pressure and reduces the risk of heart disease. The heart has considerably less work to do when pumping blood through a lean body than one with excess fat and the network of blood vessels required to feed it.

Extremely high blood pressure is a dangerous condition, and when it occurs, medications are often essential. But medications often produce undesirable side effects that lead people to stop taking them. Many people can control their blood pressure without medications when they adopt a low-fat, controlled-salt diet, particularly a vegetarian diet.

If you are on medication currently, begin the dietary changes described in this book in consultation with your doctor, so that your medication can be adjusted as needed.

Toward an Optimal Diet

I asked William Castelli if, after all his years of seeing some people develop heart disease and others remain free of it, he could say which food choices are the best. I asked, not about halfway measures, but about a truly optimal diet. "Well, vegetarians have the best diet," Castelli said. "They have the lowest rates of coronary disease of any group in the country."

As we noted above, vegetarians are better off than even the average Boston Marathon runner! Vegetarians have extraordinarily low cholesterol, HDL ratios, and correspondingly low rates of heart troubles. "Now, some people scoff at vegetarians," Castelli said, "but they have a fraction of our heart attack rate, and they have only 40 percent of our cancer rate. They outlive us. On the average, they outlive other men by about six years now. And they outlive other women by about three years."

David Nieman, D.H. Sc., has shown even higher longevity estimates. His study showed that Seventh-Day Adventist men lived an average of 12 years longer than the average population. This was not only due to their improved diet, but also because they generally avoid smoking, alcohol, and other factors which compromise health.

A vegetarian diet, of course, is becoming more and more popular. But there are different kinds of vegetarians. Some use no animal products. This group is often referred to as vegan (pronounced vee'gun). Others, often called ovo-lacto vegetarians, eat dairy products or eggs. (I have a friend who says he is pretty much a vegetarian, except that he eats eggs, dairy products, chicken, and fish—he is what we call an "ovo-lactopesco-pollo vegetarian"—in other words, not a vegetarian at all.) Ovo-lacto vegetarians do not have cholesterol levels as low as pure vegetarians.[14] Castelli found that the cardiovascular status of people on a pure vegetarian diet was excellent. Grains, legumes, vegetables, fruits, soups, and exotic sauces fill this type of menu.

But most of us were not raised as vegetarians. While we know that meat and dairy products are loaded with fat and devoid of fiber, a shift toward a meatless diet is not automatic. For some, the best way is to add a few vegetarian meals to one's routine and gradually increase the number of meatless entrees over time. For others, it helps to shift in steps—first, abandoning red meat, poultry, and fish, and later, phasing out dairy products. Castelli suggests a gradual approach. "Most families only eat from about 10 or 12 recipes. They tend to eat the same stuff night after night after night. Any time you make one of those recipes a pure vegetarian recipe, you're going to be way ahead of the game in terms of the total health impact.

"We ought to be helping people to find ways to do this. I tell them, go out and buy all the vegetarian cookbooks you can get your hands on. Try the recipes, one after another, and if you don't like it, don't feel bad, just toss it. On to the next. If you did that, you could find 10 recipes that you'd enjoy, and that would be the secret to success."

We can get plenty of protein without eating meat. "You can get good protein from cereals," Castelli said. "But what we do to cereals in this country is a crime. We take whole grain cereals, and we remove the wheat germ. We stick the wheat germ in a jar, and we sell it to you separately. We take out all the bran and shove that in a box and sell that separately. What's left over we fluff up, puff out, flake, spray on chocolate and strawberries and all this kiddy-goo stuff. And that's what we get to eat for breakfast.

"Now they're taking the bran that they took out initially, and they're spraying that back on. So we have all these new fiber-enriched cereals. The problem with some of them is that they spray on coconut oil at the same time. The reason they use coconut oil is that it's a totally saturated fat, and it resists oxidation. So the flakes stay crispier longer. The flake who ate it, however, did not stay crispier longer."

The optimal food plan, then, is a vegetarian one. Savory meals can be prepared from grains, beans, and other legumes, vegetables, and fruits. Most doctors now recognize the need to reduce meats, but will often dilute their recommendations if they believe their patients are unwilling to accept them. Unfortunately, halfway measures only work halfway. Given the power of changes in the diet, it's best to understand what an optimal diet is, and then devise a strategy that makes the change manageable, as we'll see in Chapter Nine.

The message is clear. Half of us will die of heart disease. If you have children, chances are that heart disease will eventually kill them too, unless you take preventive steps for them.

But the good news is finally here. Heart disease can be stopped. And the dietary changes that prevent or reverse heart disease also help prevent cancer, help keep our weight down, and prevent a whole host of other common problems. If we can get over a few hurdles of dietary change, we find ourselves in a whole new race. Our lives will be longer and healthier; our spouses and children—and even our parents—can be active and healthy well into a ripe old age.

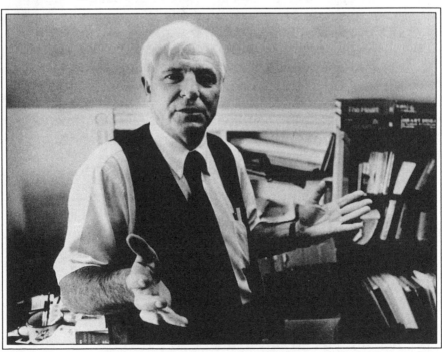

Dr. William Castelli

Tumors in the Heart?

The Research of Earl Benditt, M.D.,

of the University of Washington

What is heart disease? We know the factors that lead to it. We know what happens to those who have it. But what can we say about the disease itself? How does it begin? And how do plaques develop, the lesions which ultimately strangle the flow of blood to the heart muscle?

At the University of Washington, pathologist Earl Benditt took a close look at atherosclerosis, or common heart disease. He focused on the plaques, which are raised "bumps" on the inside walls of arteries. These plaques do not just contain fat and cholesterol; they also contain overgrown clusters of muscle cells. These muscle cells are normally found in the wall of the artery, giving it strength like the steel belts in an automobile tire. But in common heart disease, these muscle cells overgrow and burst into the artery passage to form plaques along with cholesterol and fat.

Benditt found that these cells are, in fact, the identical progeny of *a single cell* growing and multiplying out of control. Is heart disease basically a group of tumors in the artery wall, rather like cancer? Could that be why smoking contributes to heart disease just as it leads to cancer? Is that why a high-fat diet may lead to both heart disease and certain forms of cancer?

"Assuming that a plaque does derive from a single cell, then what you do is to consider the possibilities," Benditt said. "What might initiate a selective advantage for one cell type? This is precisely what happens in cancer. It looks like cancer builds in stages, and at some point a single cell appears to have gained a proliferative advantage."

What starts this process?

"Whatever it is, there has to be something. We began to explore chemical mutagens.* There appears to be an increased incidence of coronary heart disease in people who smoke, and we know perfectly well that there are lots of mutagens in cigarette smoke, the bulk of which hit the lung. If the blood levels of fats and cholesterol are up, you might expect to find more fat-soluble mutagens taken up from the lungs of cigarette smokers. We showed that certain mutagenic chemicals in cigarette smoke are carried along with the cholesterol.

"A virus is another possibility. And you can think of different ways in which the viruses can work. A virus can integrate into the genetic material of a single cell, for example, and then it becomes like a mutation."

Lowering cholesterol levels works to prevent heart disease. Whether it does so by reducing the body's tendency to form these overgrown clusters of cells or by reducing the transport of mutagenic chemicals to the artery wall is not known.

"There are so many variables that probably contribute to atherosclerosis. People speak of it as being multi-factorial, and that's a perfectly reasonable thing to do. The issue becomes how you separate the factors, how you put your finger on a factor to look at—the combination of using one's imagination, looking for analogies, and looking for things that might be related to what you're interested in, rather than simply following your prejudice."

---

*A mutagen is a substance which damages genetic material, that is, our DNA.

Chapter 2

Dr. Michael Debakey: An Interview

Michael Debakey is a pioneer in heart transplants, by-passes, and the artificial heart, and the author of countless medical publications. Although he has spent decades in the operating room undoing the damage of unhealthful dietary habits, in the past several years DeBakey has often beaten his scalpel into a plowshare, educating patients on healthier ways to eat so as to prevent the need for the operations he has developed. His recent books include *The Living Heart* and *The Living Heart Diet* (Grosset and Dunlap).

DeBakey's principal interest is in artherosclerosis, in which plaques containing cholesterol and other substances are formed in the walls of the arteries.

Although he is a demanding and meticulous researcher, he is a warm and friendly man who is generous with his time and his ideas. His dietary approach is a conservative one. He promotes a moderately low-fat diet and is concerned that patients may find greater changes unacceptable. Even so, he fondly recalls the spiced rice and beans of his Louisiana youth, which probably were far lower in fat than most "prudent" heart recipes.

Barnard: Do you feel, as a cardiovascular surgeon over so many years, that you have been working to undo the damage that people's life-styles have been doing to them?

DeBakey: We see so many cardiovascular problems that we have to deal with surgically, and then we see these same people afterwards going back to their old life-styles. You take care of their immediate complaints, and as they begin to feel normal, they slip right back into their old habits. It really is important to educate them.

> *"We see so many cadio-vascular problems that we have to deal with surgically, and then we see these same people afterwards going back to their old life-styles. It really is important to educate them."*
>
> **Dr. Michael DeBakey**

Barnard: Does that mean that a heart bypass will fail if they don't change their diet?*

DeBakey: There's no question in our minds that the risk is greater if they tend to continue with a high-fat diet.

Barnard: They develop new atherosclerosis earlier?

DeBakey: Yes, and there may be progression.

Barnard: I read that Philip Blaiberg [at one time the longest surviving heart transplant patient operated on by Dr. Christiaan Barnard] ultimately died, not from rejection, but rather from the development of new atherosclerosis because he had not changed his diet. Perhaps it was a similar situation there.

---

*The coronary arteries are those that feed the heart muscle itself. When they are blocked by plaques, the heart muscle loses part of its blood supply, causing pain and poor heart function. Obstruction of the left main coronary artery, for example, is a very critical situation. In coronary artery bypass surgery, segments of an artery or vein taken from another part of the body are placed onto the heart to provide a route for blood circulation around blocked coronary arteries to feed the heart muscle. In most cases, three arteries are bypassed in one operation.

DeBakey: There's no question that this does occur even more rapidly with heart transplants.

Barnard: People may feel that changing their diets won't help because there may be hereditary factors in heart disease.

DeBakey: It is true that a small percentage of patients have a hereditary form of arteriosclerosis in the sense that in their immediate family and their parents' and grandparents' families, there is a high incidence of atherosclerosis and coronary disease. Then, there is a form of hyper-cholesterolemia, hyperlipoproteinemia, that is definitely genetic.* But that only constitutes about five percent of the cases. So I believe that most people don't really have hereditary disease.

Barnard: It's diet and smoking?

DeBakey: Well, it's hard to say because we don't know the exact cause, and we make a point of that in our book. We frankly admit that we don't know the cause of the disease. We therefore cannot guarantee that if you follow these recommendations you're not going to have arteriosclerosis. But we do know from experience that there are three major risk factors: hyperlipidemia (cholesterol, triglycerides, and so on, are elevated), cigarette smoking, and high blood pressure. And if you can eliminate those three, it has been clearly demonstrated statistically over a period of time that the incidence will be reduced.

Barnard: Is there a time when a person is too old to benefit from changing the diet?

DeBakey: No, we don't think so. We strongly recommend to people in their sixties and even in their seventies that I operate on, to go on a definite dietary regimen. And if they've been on a high-fat content diet, we strongly urge them to reduce the fat content to maybe 20 to 30 percent.

Barnard: In *The Living Heart Diet*, you point out that 60 to 80 percent of cholesterol is manufactured by the body.

DeBakey: Yes.

---

*Hypercholesterolemia is an elevated cholesterol level in the blood, one of the main risk factors for heart disease. Hyperlipoproteinemia means high levels of lipoproteins, the packages that deliver cholesterol.

Barnard: That would suggest that there is a limit to what dietary changes can accomplish.

DeBakey: Actually dietary changes can accomplish quite a bit. Let's say you have a cholesterol level of 250. If you go on a strict dietary regimen in which you reduce your fat content to below 30 percent of your total diet, you will definitely reduce the cholesterol level in your blood. Now, if you took zero fat in your diet, you will definitely reduce the cholesterol level in your blood. Now, if you took zero fat in your diet, you're still going to make cholesterol out of whatever you eat, if you live. Cholesterol is an essential component of life. So we're not talking about that part. We're talking about the excess.

> *"We strongly recommend to people in their sixties and even in their seventies that I operate on, to go on a definite dietary regimen. And if they've been on a high-fat content diet, we strongly urge them to reduce the fat content to maybe 20 to 30 percent."*
>
> **Dr. Michael DeBakey**

Barnard: You mention in this book that one of the mechanisms of reducing cholesterol is that fiber in the diet binds cholesterol that the body secretes in the form of bile salts and allows it to be excreted before it can be reabsorbed.

DeBakey: That's right.

Barnard: In your own experience, does the availability of coronary artery bypass surgery decrease patients' motivation for preventive measures.

DeBakey: I don't think it does, at least in my experience. I operated on a patient today, for example. This was his third bypass in fifteen years. He came back for his second bypass about six or seven years ago. And he did fine until about six months ago, when he started having more pain. And it got worse and worse.

Two of his three bypasses were blocked. I operated on him today. I did not only those two that were blocked, but also the other one because the vein was beginning to show some thickening. Now this patient has done as well as he could have on his regimen. His cholesterol wasn't elevated. He quit smoking a long time ago and has never smoked since. Blood pressure has been under good control. He just happens to be one of those people who belongs in that category of patients in whom atherosclerosis develops no matter what. And, interestingly, 40 to 50 percent of patients will have no risk factors.

Barnard: If he lowered the fat in his diet to well below the 30 percent you recommend in your book, to as close as possible to the zero level you mentioned, would he do better?

DeBakey: He might. I don't know. One of the reasons that we don't eliminate all fat from the diet is that it's very difficult to stay on such a diet. You take these very radical diets that are advocated from time to time. Nobody can stay on them. That's why they are unsuccessful. It's not that they're not effective immediately. But nobody would want to remain on that kind of diet. And that's why our menus are all low-fat, but there's some fat in the diet. You have to make the food taste good.

Barnard: So, in other words, your recipes aren't necessarily the healthiest ones, but they're the ones you think are most likely to be accepted?

DeBakey: No, not necessarily. The menus in our book provide a healthy diet. We give all kinds of data so that the person can learn something about nutrition. The menus include desserts like pastries (margarine pastry), honey apple pie, cherry nut pie, banana oatmeal cookies, brownies

Barnard: I notice *The Living Heart Diet* also includes international foods, beans and rice, for example, which I suppose most people here don't eat, but in Mexico or other countries are much more common.

DeBakey: Yes. We have them here, and they're good. People in certain parts of the country, like my part of the country, south Louisiana where I was born and reared, eat rice every day. Bean dishes are also popular. Beans were formerly considered poor man's food. We have several menus in the book for beans and rice that are delicious. I've had them myself, and my wife, who is a good cook, has used them and likes them. There are rice recipes in the book that are quite good: brown rice, white rice, enriched rice, with and without salt, and so on.

If rice is prepared properly, it's very tasty. The trouble is most people think of rice the way the Chinese prepare it. They like it that way, but we prepare rice with something else, so that the rice is not just boiled. It can be mixed with herbs to make it very tasty. Rice and beans are good foods.

Barnard: Good for longevity. How have you avoided coronary artery disease in your own life? Are you jogging every morning?

DeBakey: No, I don't jog.

Barnard: I don't get the impression you take many vacations, looking at the list of articles and books you've written.

DeBakey: No, I don't take vacations. I do a lot of travelling, both in the States and overseas. I just returned from Australia. I went to Chicago this past week. Next week I'm going to Costa Rica. In a couple of weeks I have to go to Europe. Because I do so much traveling, I don't take formal vacations. And because I'm active all the time, I don't take formal exercise; I usually try to use the stairs here. I walk up and down these stairs from the operating room, which is six floors down. So that gives me a bit of exercise. I maintain a pretty active program. And I'm a very moderate eater.

Barnard: In terms of quantity?

DeBakey: Yes. I love vegetables and fruits. I really have only one meal a day, usually in the evening when I go home.

Barnard: No breakfast or lunch usually?

DeBakey: A piece of fruit.

Barnard: A piece of fruit for breakfast.

DeBakey: And lunch may be just yogurt or something like that. Lunch for me is not a specific time because of my operating schedule. I don't know what time I'll be out of the operating room. I may be out at ten or I may not be out until three.

Barnard: How about children? Children love ice cream, they love McDonald's. Should they be taught differently from an early age?

DeBakey: Yes. I think so. We've done that in our family with my children. I have an eight-year old daughter, and she's never eaten anything at a fast-food restaurant.

Barnard: Your daughter has never been to McDonald's?

DeBakey: Well, she has gone to such places with some of her friends, but because my wife and I have strongly urged her not to eat any fast foods, she will go in with her friends maybe for a little bit, but she won't eat anything. She's never had a hamburger from those places because we don't want her eating that kind of food. We want her to learn to like the kind of food that we have on the table.

We are doing a program for children—teaching the parents and the children. You have to educate the parents first. You can't teach the children without having educated parents. So we have a program in which the parents and the children are being taught how to control their diet. There is more to it than just fat content. Nutrition is the key word. That's why they have to understand what nutrition is.

Barnard: Can the schools play a part too?

DeBakey: Absolutely. In fact, we're working with the schools on this.

Barnard: I wonder about this in the hospitals. When I go in the hospital cafeteria, they've got a lot of nice developments, but they're all toward making the food more attractive. They have a dessert bar and so on.

DeBakey: You're quite right about that. I don't know the reason for it. I suppose the cafeteria is a section of some department and they hire cooks and leave it at their discretion, but the cafeteria should be under the control of a good nutritionist.

Barnard: Many hospital nutritionists in my experience are still saying a lot of outdated things—the old "four food groups" and so on.

DeBakey: You're right.

Barnard: Some probably wouldn't like your own dietary habits and would counsel you to have more meat in your diet and so on. I think it's appalling.

DeBakey: Yes, I agree. I don't eat in the cafeteria here, and I don't know what kind of cafeteria we have. I hope it's not that bad. I just got back from Illinois, and although I didn't eat in the cafeteria, we went through to get a cup of coffee, and I saw what they had. You're absolutely correct.

Barnard: I imagine you may have had better influence here than we have there.

DeBakey: Well, yes, we have. That's why we have this restaurant we call Chez Eddy. If you get a chance to go there and have a meal, you ought to. The food is delightfully prepared, beautifully presented, and very well controlled as far as nutrition is concerned.

Barnard: You mention in *The Living Heart Diet* that atherosclerosis has some similarities to cancer, based on Earl Benditt's research in Seattle. The muscle cells which reinforce the artery wall start to overgrow to form plaques, which are very much like tumors.

DeBakey: That's right.

Barnard: Since the sex hormones that fuel cancer of the breast, prostate, and other organs are made from cholesterol, is there a connection between heart disease and cancer or is that a coincidence?

DeBakey: We don't know. That hypothesis of Benditt and his group is very appealing. I personally feel there has to be something that starts it off. That's one reason that we have been doing some work with the hospitals here looking into a virus.

We have now published two papers on this study. Dr. [Joseph L.] Melnick, who is one of the great experts in virology, is working with us. We take specimens from patients and give them to him to study; he has clearly demonstrated a herpetic type of virus associated with atherosclerosis. What we don't know is whether that's just a part of everybody having that virus or whether it has some definite relation to the atheroma.

Barnard: So the key would be to have some control patients who had had traumatic deaths for comparison.

DeBakey: That's right. We're continuing that research.

Barnard: What is the current advice on polyunsaturates? We've heard you should have more; others say all fats should be greatly reduced because they promote cancer.

DeBakey: It's hard to say. Because of epidemiologic studies, I would tend to reduce the total amount too. The body's going to make what you need. So why give it an excess in the foods you're consuming? Eat only the amount you need to make the food taste good. A certain amount of fat is inherent in the preparation of foods, but keep it to a minimum.

Barnard: How did Americans get on this diet we're on that seems to be so destructive?

DeBakey: I think to some extent it's simply due to the fact that our country's so much better off economically. You don't see this kind of a diet in poor countries where the economic level of the people is low. They eat very little red meat because meat is too expensive. Now the fast-food chains have centered on hamburgers, filled with oil that they're cooked in, with french fries also cooked in oil. It's largely, I think, the economic development of the people in this country that has created that kind of a diet. The Western Europeans are similarly affluent. But the diets of South and Central Americans, Africans, Indians, and Chinese contain little fat and little meat, and they're better off for it.

Barnard: You mention in *The Living Heart Diet* that cholesterol is mainly in the lean portion of meat. Trimming the fat helps, but most of the cholesterol will still be there.

DeBakey: Yes, that's why you have to control the amount. Restaurants serve you a tremendous steak—too much for one person. I don't order steak. If I'm at a banquet or some place where I don't have an opportunity to order, I usually don't eat much of what is served.

Barnard: After all the things you've accomplished as a physician, the innovations you've brought to medicine, what are your gratifications in your work?

DeBakey: My gratification comes from my work—daily activities. Each morning I get up and have a full schedule ahead of me of things to do. It's gratifying to know that some of the things you've done are accepted and perhaps you've received honors for, but you don't live on that. Those are gratifying, I must say. They give you some reassurance about what you've done. But you live every day. As far as I'm concerned, I do the best I can each day to enjoy the work that I'm doing. Sometimes there are heartbreaks. It's not all ecstasy, you know. There's some agony in it too. But my gratification really comes in doing it, or trying to do it anyway.

Barnard: Solving clinical problems.

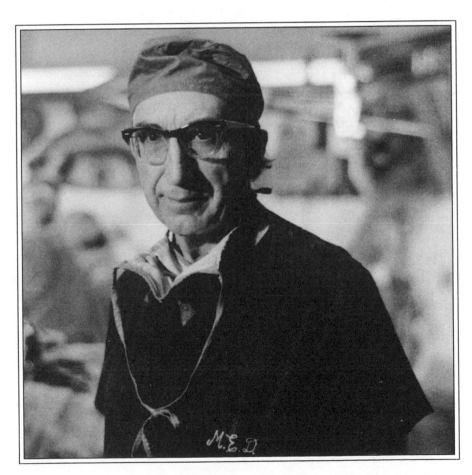

Dr. Michael DeBakey

DeBakey: Yes.

Barnard: What's ahead in terms of your own practice and research interests?

DeBakey: Arteriosclerosis/atherosclerosis is my main concern, and the one I'm giving the most attention to. Some of it is clinical in the sense that we're trying to assess what I've done clinically, so I follow my patients. I have records that I'm analyzing all the time. And some is more research-oriented, in perhaps developing ways to deal with certain problems that we have not yet solved, particularly end-stage heart disease. We are trying to find out if there is some way we can open up arteries that are clogged all the way. So we're doing both clinical and experimental work in various areas.

Barnard: How is the work developing for end-stage patients?

DeBakey: I would say for end-stage coronary disease, I suppose cardiac transplantation right now is the best. We're getting about an 85 percent first-year survival rate and projecting a 50 percent five-year survival rate. And it may be closer to 60 percent five-year survival. So, right now that's the only answer we have. The trouble is, of course, that that's limited because you have limitations on the donor. At least 40 to 50 percent of patients that we consider candidates for a transplant die before we can find a donor.

Barnard: Can we reduce the number who need them?

DeBakey: That's one of the things we're working on—trying to find ways to do this. The trouble is that I'm not sure that even if you restored circulation to some of these, the muscle would come back.

Barnard: The heart muscle is so deteriorated from poor circulation?

DeBakey: Yes. We do have some evidence that if we get them early enough, before the damage has existed for a long time, we can restore muscular function, with improvement in the patient. And we have evidence that the ejection fractions and muscular function are improved.*

---

*Ejection fraction is a measure of how effectively blood is pumped by the heart.

But if the damage is extended beyond a certain point, there's not much chance to restore the circulation.

Barnard: So, for typical atherosclerotic heart disease, if they're not bypassed early on—

DeBakey: Or the artery is not opened up by some other means, like balloon angioplasty or lysis of the clot, if it is blocked by a clot.

Barnard: So, if there's no early surgical intervention, then there's nothing else to be done other than a heart transplant?

DeBakey: Not in all patients, because in some the heart still has sufficient function to pump adequately for some time after a heart attack. I'm talking about when the heart reaches that stage where the ejection fraction is down to 20 or less. Very little can be done at that stage to improve it.

Barnard: What are the current indications for bypass? I know it's been a heated controversy. Some say it doesn't prolong life.

DeBakey: In certain forms of heart disease, I don't think it's any better than medical treatment because the disease is too mild.

Barnard: Where only one or two of the coronary arteries are involved?

DeBakey: Yes. But in other forms, three vessels are involved and their function has been somewhat impaired; if the patient is operated on early enough, his condition will improve. I also think the survival rate is better than with medical treatment.

Barnard: So it does more than decrease angina, that is, chest pain.

DeBakey: Angina is just one manifestation of the disease. For example, this patient that I operated on this morning for the third time. We certainly didn't want to operate on him. When you're operating in this area the third time, you have a big technical problem, and you increase the risk of operation considerably. I explained all that to this man, and he said, "Well, what else could I have?" I Said, "The only other treatment we have is medical." And he replied,

"I've been on that six weeks, and I'm not any better. You got any better medical treatment?" And we said, "No, that's the best medical treatment we can give you." And he said, "Well, I can't live like this. I can't walk half a block. I wake up three, four, or five times during the night and take nitroglycerine." He said, "I just don't want to live this way. I'll take whatever risk there is, so that can be improved." So pain can often be a very important factor. It it's uncontrollable by medical means then surgical treatment is indicated.

But that's not the only indication. There are others—sometimes when pain is not a big factor but limitation of activity is. Then we see some patients who, for example, have very critical disease like left main obstruction. And I have patients who have not only left main obstruction, but stenosis of the right coronary artery. Those people can die of a sudden heart attack any moment. So, I think the indications are largely the severity of disease, the severity of symptoms which are uncontrollable medically, and anatomic disease that jeopardizes the patient's life.

Barnard: Some people have claimed that heart bypasses do not prolong life. The Coronary Artery Surgery Study (CASS), for example, has been used as evidence that, at least in mild forms of heart disease, bypasses do no good at all.[1]

DeBakey: Unfortunately, a certain amount of misleading information has been disseminated. The misleading information came, to a large extent, from news reports, including even *60 Minutes*, but the medical profession is also responsible, not because the report was inaccurate, but because the impression the report gave was inaccurate, and then it was quoted inaccurately. I'm referring to the so-called CASS study. If you read the CASS study itself, there was nothing inaccurate about it. It was quite correct. But the study was done on a very small subset of patients with coronary disease. In other words, it took nearly 30,000 patients that they reviewed in order to get—

Barnard: 700 and some for the study.

DeBakey: Yes, about 700 patients with this very mild form of coronary disease. In fact, we were asked to participate in the study when they originally came out with it six or seven years ago. And we said no, we couldn't ethically do it, because we had already decided at that time those patients should not be operated on.

Barnard: So they were operating on people who didn't need it.

DeBakey: That's exactly right; they were operating on people who didn't need it. And we felt that was unethical. And in my commentary on the study, which was published in *JAMA*, I pointed that out.[2] Well, the news media didn't do anything else but take that study and never qualified it. They just said "all patients with angina and coronary disease." They didn't say this was a very small subset of a very mild form of disease. They didn't say there are many doctors who weren't operating on them when they started the study. Even worse, they got statisticians to say that on that basis, 25,000 patients were being operated on unnecessarily.

Barnard: Making a scandal.

DeBakey: Yes. And the worst one was *60 Minutes*. This fellow, Mike Wallace, came down here and spent a day with me. Never put me on. He completely edited my remarks out of the program because I told the truth about it and gave him a copy of my commentary. But that didn't fit in with their notion about what they wanted to do to make it controversial.

Barnard: Your commentary is rather straightforward and clear. Why didn't they find it compelling?

DeBakey: *60 Minutes*? Because that wasn't what they wanted. What they wanted to say was 25,000 people were being operated on unnecessarily. When the truth doesn't fit in with their notions of what is presentable, they don't include it.

What is interesting is that they took the other patients from the CASS study for whom they had records, some of whom had been operated on and others hadn't. They didn't do the same study they did with this small number, but they got follow-ups on them. They've come out with a series of articles clearly demonstrating that in three-vessel disease and in patients with impaired function (damage), operation has proved to be better than medical treatment.

Barnard: If everyone reads your book and does what you do with your own family, you may be finding a lot fewer patients for bypass surgery.

DeBakey: Yes, I think it will reduce the number. Somebody estimated—I have no reason to confirm or deny this estimate—that if these risk factors were closely followed and people really paid attention to their diet, weight, and other preventive measures, we could reduce the incidence by 30 percent.

Barnard: The incidence of bypasses?

DeBakey: The incidence of coronary disease. Surely that would include bypasses as well. And I must say, I'm inclined to believe that.

Barnard: Could we reduce it more through even more dietary modification?

DeBakey: I don't think we will be able to reduce it significantly beyond that point until we know the cause. All we're doing is hitting at some of these factors that contribute but don't cause it. That's why it's so important to find the cause.

Barnard: How are we doing in that regard?

DeBakey: I think we have a ways to go. We know a lot more about it—the pathogenesis, the way it forms, and all sorts of things. But what is the initial cause? There's always something that causes a disease. Once it's found, it's specific, whether it's a virus or a bacteria or some kind of deficiency—hormone or vitamin or whatever. It's always specific.

Barnard: What are the studies we should be pushing in that regard?

DeBakey: It's very difficult to say. I personally believe that the more basic biologic studies, understanding the biology at the cellular level, work along the lines that Benditt and groups of that kind are doing, and some of the work we're doing with viruses and so on, will give us a better understanding of the disease.

Barnard: Let me follow up on what you were saying about heart transplants. How do we deal with the lack of availability of hearts?

DeBakey: Mostly, I think, by trying to educate the public to be more understanding and therefore to give permission. Probably part of the problem is that it's always a tragedy, and the potential donor is relatively young. Young healthy people don't usually die of disease. They die from accidents, and it's always tragic and sudden. The last transplant I did was about five or six days ago. The donor was a 17-year-old boy who shot himself. A tragedy. We had another donor, also a 17-year-old boy who was playing with his friends, and he happened to be sitting on a car that was moving, not rapidly, but he fell off and hit his head some way and had brain death. It's very difficult at that point to talk to the family to get them to give permission. So we have to educate the public, and I think this is being done, but right now we're only reaching about 30 percent of available donors.

Barnard: What do you think of the proposals for animal donors?

DeBakey: It is not feasible right now because we simply don't have a way of controlling the rejection adequately. Cross-species rejection is so severe, and there's not much chance right now of controlling it. It may be possible some day, when we have a better understanding of some of the genetics involving the immune mechanism of the body— to modify that without destroying the whole immune function.

Barnard: So when Leonard Bailey put a baboon heart into Baby Fae—

DeBakey: The baby never had a chance.

Barnard: He says it's because he failed to match the blood types.

DeBakey: It wouldn't have made any difference.

Barnard: I guess what was disturbing was that there was the Norwood repair procedure that might have been done for her hypoplastic left heart.

DeBakey: Yes. He obviously was determined to do it. And I questioned him at a symposium on transplants and implants that I was asked to moderate in Louisville. He wasn't on the program. He just appeared and asked for time to present his experience. And I said, "Surely." I questioned him about the incident rather sharply. I asked him to give any evidence that would provide support for doing the procedure. And he said the evidence was his own experimental work. I asked, "What reports have you published?" He replied that they hadn't been published yet. And I said, "Can you give a summary of what you found?" And he did. I said, "Did you have any long-term survivors at all?" His reply was "No."

Barnard: In the animal work?

DeBakey: Yes, he did cross-animal work. Cross-species. Anyway, he said he thought a baby—an infant at that stage—the immune mechanism was not very strong, hadn't been developed well. And he thought with cyclosporine he might be able to hold off until he could find a donor. And I said, "Did you look for a donor first?" He said he didn't. I asked if he planned to do it anyway. And he admitted that he did. I really think that what he did does not have adequate scientific basis. I doubt seriously if you'll see it repeated.

Barnard: I understand this was only the first of a series of five they'd planned to do. Perhaps they're concerned that that might lead to some legal troubles.

DeBakey: I don't know. They've been criticized for it.

Barnard: This brings up the whole question of animals in research. You know, we had a flap about this at the military medical school in Bethesda, Maryland, the Uniformed Services University of the Health Sciences. They were going to shoot dogs to teach debridement, that is, the "cleaning up" of gunshot wounds. I ask you this also because of your wartime experience. The argument the military makes is that a high-velocity wound looks so different from a typical gunshot wound that you have to practice on animals. But I should think debridement principles would apply to all wounds.

DeBakey: No, the trouble is that there is a difference. There's no question about it. We learned that in World War II. The question is whether you need to shoot animals to teach physicians how to debride wounds. I'm not really sure that's necessary. I'm one of the consultants at the Uniformed

Services University, and I understand some of their concerns and some of the things they're trying to learn about high-velocity wounds—the extent to which damage is done beyond the surrounding area. Some research is needed in that area. But I think it has to be very specific.

Barnard: I think we, ourselves, have to cut out those uses of animals that are clearly unnecessary. For example, when I was in medical school we didn't learn blood-drawing (venipuncture) on animals. We learned it on the guy in the next desk. I learned to intubate on a patient.

DeBakey: I agree with you. I don't think we would learn that sort of thing on animals in our institution. We teach them how to do these things—venipuncture, intubation, gastric tubes—on humans because we're doing them on humans.

Barnard: Cutdowns, chest tubes, and so on?

DeBakey: Yes. We have to do them on humans to treat them. Why shouldn't the student learn on humans? I gave up surgical training of our students and residents on animals years ago. We used to have a course. I stopped it completely. I said, "I'm not going to do this anymore on animals because we're going to put students in the operating room with humans."

Barnard: How about teaching the techniques of vascular surgery or open heart surgery?

DeBakey: You don't have to have a living animal to try to do microsurgery, say to repair a vessel. You can use fresh cadavers. It's very easy. You just take a piece of tissue out of a fresh cadaver, whether it's an animal that died from some other reason or a human.

Barnard: Is that how you train the residents here—cadavers?

DeBakey: Yes.

Barnard: And I guess the operating room is a place for a kind of apprenticeship for residents, where they can observe and gradually take over under supervision.

DeBakey: Absolutely. A lot can be done if one thinks.

Barnard: As opposed to—

DeBakey: Well, as opposed to accepting some tradition or previous way of doing things without thinking about it.

Chapter 3

Tackling
Cancer

There is a way to beat cancer. It is not found in the newspapers generally. Every press release of a "breakthrough" drowns in the wave of ever-increasing death rates. But there is a new approach. We now know that the vast majority of cancers *can actually be prevented.*

Time For A New Strategy

"CANCER TESTS: FLOOD OF HOPE,
AN EXCITING FIRST STEP"

read the headline of *USA Today.* Eleven patients with advanced cancer had improved. One had had a complete disappearance of the disease. The miracle drug was interleukin 2. The miracle worker was a researcher at the National Cancer Institute. Calls flooded in. Dying patients and their relatives seized on the hope that, at the eleventh hour, long after hopes carefully constructed between doctor and patient had been bitterly relinquished in the onslaught of cancer, at last, the long-awaited cure was here. The doctor looked clean and confident in the accompanying picture. One patient, a father of five, had faced a certain death from advanced skin cancer. But now he felt "hopeful for the future. There are visible signs I'm getting well. I'm excited. My whole family is excited. I don't know why we've been so blessed."

But it was not to be, at least, not yet. He died six months after the *USA Today* article appeared. No patient on the interleukin 2 treatment had been cured. It was not a silver bullet. Barely a year after the media burst, a harsh editorial in the *Journal of the American Medical Association* (*JAMA*) stated "One would . . . hope that investigators will suppress the urge to publicly state or imply that a breakthrough has taken place until solid evidence exists . . ."[1] Interleukin 2 seemed to be little better than other chemotherapies. It was also extraordinarily poisonous. The editorial called the treatment "an awesome experience" with "devastating toxic reactions" and "astronomical costs." The researchers acknowledged that interleukin 2 was "very toxic . . . very cumbersome and very expensive" and that it had contributed to the deaths of four patients.

Interleukin 2 had followed on the heels of alpha-interferon and other anti-cancer drugs which were widely hailed, only to prove disappointing. "We are definitely not winning with respect to treatment," says cancer researcher John Bailar, M.D., Ph.D. Bailar had been a career researcher at the National Cancer Institute (NCI), and for years was Editor in Chief of the *Journal of the National Cancer Institute*. He had slowly and carefully gone through the figures of what the War on Cancer had—and had not—accomplished. We are losing—losing more patients than ever, losing this medical Vietnam, a war in which we lack the vision we need to win.

> *"There have been some very important advances in cancer treatment. But with respect to the cure of cancer, they are limited largely to perhaps one or two percent of the total cancer burden."*
>
> **Dr. John Bailar**

John Bailar is a large man. Sporting a moustache and shirt sleeves, he appears surprisingly casual for one of the leaders in cancer research. He has the sturdy look of a Teddy Roosevelt with a kind demeanor and professorial patience.

"There have been some very important advances in cancer treatment over the last three decades," Bailar said. "But with respect to the cure of cancer, they are limited largely to the cancers that tend to occur in children and young adults, and those make up only perhaps one or two percent of the total cancer burden."

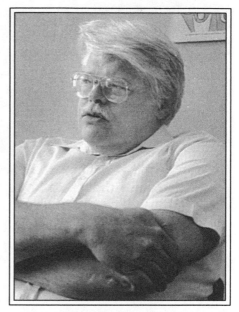

Unfortunately, we have only managed to impact on the more rare malignancies with little effect on the most common and deadly forms of cancer. There have been some advances in alleviating cancer, but cures for the most common cancers, unfortunately, remain out of reach.

"Cancer death rates continue to go up year after year," Bailar said. "Now, these are real increases. I've taken out the effect of the changing size of the popu-

Dr. John Bailar

lation, the changing age structure, declining mortality from other diseases, and we look at what's left. There is a genuine increase in the frequency of deaths from cancer, and this has been going on quite steadily for a number of years now."

Like the bad news given by a doctor to a cancer patient, his message was met with hostility and defensiveness by many with a stake in research for cancer treatments. But further studies have shown precisely the same thing.

Lung cancer is going up because of tobacco; cancer treatments can do little to stem the death toll. Bailar states, "There is a long lead time between the initiation of smoking as a regular habit and the appearance of lung cancer," Bailar said. "It may be twenty, thirty, forty years or more for some people. So, what we're seeing now is the effect of the rise in tobacco use several decades ago. I think that in years to come we'll see the effect of the curtailing of smoking that is going on now. It just takes a long time to do this."

For breast and prostate cancer, the death rates are not improving. For colorectal cancer, there is a gradual decline, but it is quite slow. Stomach cancer and cervical cancer are occurring *less* often, but when they do occur, treatment is essentially no more effective now than it was decades ago. Year after year, these diseases take a tremendous toll. It is not that researchers are not trying. They simply are not succeeding.

"The degree of improvement in death rates in general for the common cancers of adults is really pretty discouraging," Bailar said. "It has not been for lack of effort. We have poured vast amounts of money into the search for cancer cures over a very long period of time. We've brought some of the best research minds we have to bear on these problems, and it just hasn't worked."

Eighty Percent Preventable

Instead of struggling—and failing—to cure cancer after it has developed, can we prevent it from occurring in the first place? If cancer is caused by environmental or life-style factors, then it potentially can be prevented. In fact, the National Cancer Institute estimates that as much as eighty percent of cancer cases theoretically can be prevented. Some estimates are even higher.

> *"The degree of improvement in death rates in general for the common cancers of adults is really pretty discouraging. We have poured vast amounts of money into the search for cancer cures over a very long period of time, and it just hasn't worked."*
>
> *Dr. John Bailar*

Thirty percent of cancers are due to tobacco. Avoid smoking, and lung cancer becomes very unlikely. Federal support of tobacco crops could be ended. Unfortunately, attempts to do so have been consistently blocked by Congressmen from tobacco-growing states.

Another example is radiation. Radon is a natural radioactive gas that seeps up from certain underground rocks into groundwater supplies. Tight insulation, which has been more widely used as fuel costs have risen, causes radon to build up in enclosed areas. Improved ventilation helps bring these levels back down. But the most potent area for prevention is diet. When researchers have examined the factors responsible for increased cancer risk, dietary changes are at the top of the list. Thirty to sixty percent of cancers are due to dietary factors, particularly the amount of fat consumed (which increases risk) and the amounts of fiber and certain vitamins and minerals (which decrease risk).

In 1982, the National Research Council released a technical report, *Diet, Nutrition, and Cancer*, showing that diet was probably the greatest single factor in the epidemic of cancer, particularly for cancers of the breast, colon, and prostate.[2] Since then, evidence for effects of certain foods on the incidence of other types of cancer has also steadily accumulated.

Estimated Percentages of Cancer Due to Selected Factors	
Tobacco	30%
Diet	30-60%
Alcohol	3%
Radiation	3%
Air and Water Pollution	1-5%
Medications	2%

These figures are rough estimates based on data from Cancer Rates and Risks. *1985. National Cancer Institute. Washington, D.C.: Doll R, Peto R. Journal of the National Cancer Institute 1981; 66(6):1191-1308; and Alabaster, O. 1986. The Power of Prevention. Washington, D.C.: Saville Books.*

Genetic and occupational factors, sunlight, and viruses also play a role in certain forms of cancer and are not included in this table. Categories may overlap. For example, both tobacco and alcohol contribute to esophageal cancer.

A Look at Specific Foods

Dietary changes are the light at the end of the tunnel for those looking for a way to reduce the cancer epidemic. By avoiding foods that lead to cancer and including foods that strengthen us against the disease, we can, to a great extent, control our own risk.

Fats and Oils

Foods rich in fats and oils increase our cancer risk. Americans certainly eat a lot of fat. About 40 percent of all the calories we eat come from the fat in meats, poultry, fish, dairy products, fried foods, and vegetable oils. Of the many forms of cancer promoted by a high-fat diet, probably the best-studied is breast cancer. A major study by Bruce Armstrong and Richard Doll compared countries with varying diets and found a strong correlation between the per capita consumption of fat and the breast cancer rate.[3]

"Japanese women have the lowest breast cancer rate in the world," said Oliver Alabaster, M.D. "Many Japanese women have migrated to Hawaii and to the U.S. mainland. While marrying within their own community and keeping the population relatively unchanged genetically, they shifted their diet toward a more Western, higher-fat diet, and their breast cancer rate steadily climbed. Within one generation it approximated that of Caucasian women living around them. This is very dramatic evidence that cancer is mainly environmentally induced, rather than genetically inherited." And within Japan, women of high socioeconomic strata who eat meat daily have more than eight times the risk of breast cancer compared to poorer women who rarely consume meat.[4] The most likely culprit is the fat in the meat.

Alabaster is Director of the Institute for Disease Prevention at the George Washington University Medical Center. Alabaster knows about breast cancer; he lost his own mother to the disease. Her cancer was diagnosed at the age of 41. She had a mastectomy and radiation treatments, the standard techniques at the time. But seven years after diagnosis, she succumbed to the advancing illness.

Alabaster was the first to write a simple, convincing guide for the layman on how to prevent cancer. *The Power of Prevention* (Saville Books, 1986) shows how to take one's risk in hand and actually change it. In reviewing the evidence, he became convinced that fat in the diet was a major contributor to breast cancer, an opinion shared by the National Cancer Institute.

"There is a great deal of evidence that fat increases cancer risk," agrees Peter Greenwald, Director of Cancer Prevention and Control of the National Cancer Institute. "Certainly for breast cancer, when people move from one country to another their risk changes, and the only solid explanation that we have relates to dietary fat. We have a number of case-control epidemiologic studies consistent with this effect. There's a lot of evidence."

The differences in breast cancer rates across various countries are not due to industrialization or air pollution or stress, as Greenwald points out. "There are industrial countries like Japan with low colon and breast cancer rates," he said. "It's not just being industrialized that gives you the high cancer rate. There are rural countries such as New Zealand that have Western habits, and they have the higher cancer rate."

The problem is dietary, particularly the amount of fat we consume. "Fat" in this context refers to all types of fats— animal fats and vegetable oils. Where do we get all this fat? Meats, poultry, fish, whole milk and other dairy products, oily salad dressings, margarine, and fried foods are all sources. Even supposedly "lean meats" contain significant amounts of fat. That goes for chicken and fish as well. The leanest beef is 29 percent fat, as a percentage of calories. Skinless chicken white meat is about 23 percent fat. Fish vary from a low of about 8 percent for cod to well over 50 percent for mackerel, herring, and some types of salmon. Most fish are in the range of 20-30 percent fat. But beans are only four percent fat. Rice is only 1 percent fat. And no plant foods contain any cholesterol. "If you look at the constituents of poultry and fish, they both contain fat," Alabaster said. "It's not as if you're getting on a fat-free diet by eating poultry and fish. They still contain fat, and they contain cholesterol. Fish and poultry are the safest forms of meat, but yet they're still totally different from vegetables, whole grain cereals, fruits, and so on. Breads, cereals, fruits, and vegetables contribute very little fat, a lot of fiber, and no cholesterol. It's only what you then add which is contributing the fat and cholesterol: oils, meats, including fish and poultry for that matter, or dairy products."

That does not mean that everything that comes from plants is low in fat. Fried vegetable foods can absorb enormous amounts of fat in the process of frying. Potato chips and french fries are filled with it. For years, doctors have advocated increasing the amounts of vegetable oil in the diet to replace artery-clogging animal fat. But it is now clear that all types of fat—animal and vegetable—should be reduced. Currently, about 40 percent of the calories in the American diet comes from fat. This should be cut to about 10 percent.

How fat in the diet leads to cancer is still poorly understood. Fat is known to affect the activity of sex hormones, which, in turn, may promote certain forms of cancer. Low-fat and vegetarian diets are known to reduce the levels of female sex hormones in the blood stream, particularly estradiol, one of the naturally occurring estrogens which regulate the reproductive cycle.[5,6] Women on high-fat diets tend to have higher levels of these hormones. Sex hormones are known to promote cancer of the breast and the reproductive organs. These observations also suggest a reason behind the young age of puberty in countries where a high-fat diet is consumed. A century or two ago, puberty in girls occurred at about age seventeen. In rural Asian and African countries puberty still occurs in the later teens.[7] But in America and other Westernized societies in the past several decades, the increasing amounts of fat in the diet have been accompanied by the gradual drop in the age of puberty, probably because of abnormal elevations of sex hormones.

In addition, cancer-causing chemicals in the environment tend to dissolve into fatty tissues. Fat may also affect the ability of carcinogens to get into cells. But the situation is rather like that for tobacco. It is clear that tobacco causes cancer, but exactly how it does so is not at all clear. What is clear, for both tobacco and fat, is the need to reduce one's exposure to the offending agent.

When Japan's breast cancer rate was at its lowest, the Japanese diet was about 10 percent fat. Westernization has pushed Japan's fat intake up to 25 percent in recent decades, and breast cancer rates have steadily climbed. The National Academy of Sciences makes the modest recommendation that our fat intake be cut to 30 percent of calories. "The Academy figure was arrived at as a compromise because some thought if you make it too low nobody's going to follow it," Alabaster said. "I would argue that if you don't make it low enough, it's so worthless that you discredit the principle. There are countries where the dietary fat intake is 30 percent or 35 percent which still have high cancer rates, so I think it's a totally worthless target to lower fat only to 30 percent. You've got to go down at least to 20 percent. I wouldn't make any big issue between 15, 20, or 25 percent. Nobody knows the precise amount."

There is evidence that Alabaster was right. In 1992, a study was reported by Dr. Walter Willett and his colleagues at Harvard of a large group of nurses who had varying levels of fat in their diets. During a period of eight years, a 30-percent level of fat did not lower their risk of breast cancer at all. Reducing fat in the diet does not help, some thought. On closer inspection, one draws an entirely different conclusion. The traditional diet of people in Asia, who so rarely develop cancer, contains only about half that amount. However, support for even modest reductions come from an Italian study which showed that women whose diets derived less than 28 percent of their calories from fat had significantly less risk of breast cancer compared to women whose diets contained more than 36 percent fat.[8] Diets rich in fat, saturated fat, or animal protein were associated with a risk for cancer that was two to three times greater than normal.

Many organs that are controlled by sex hormones are affected by fat intake. The risk of cancer of these organs is related to the fat content of the diet. Breast cancer, cancers of the uterus and cervix, and in men, prostate cancer fall into this category.

Evidence has also linked fat intake to cancers of the digestive system: colon, rectum, stomach, liver, and pancreas. Fat promotes cancer, and fiber is, to an extent, protective.

Fiber

It is ironic that fiber—the part of the diet which is defined by its indigestibility—should show such power in maintaining our health. But it certainly does. The critical scientific work which established the value of fiber was done by Denis Burkitt, M.D. In his twenty years of surgical practice in Africa, Burkitt wondered why diseases which were so common in England and America were almost never encountered in Africa. The critical factor, he found, was fiber. Fiber passes undigested through the small intestine. It acts to speed the passage of food and to remove harmful substances. The refining processes of developed countries remove the fiber from grains, leading to a high incidence of several diseases. Burkitt found a particularly important connection between fiber and cancer of the colon and rectum.

> *"Of all cancers, colon cancer is the one which is most characteristic of modern Western culture. Colorectal cancer is always rare amongst primitive people. Everything points to diet, and the most important things in diet are fat and fiber."*
>
> ***Dr. Dennis Burkitt***

"Of all cancers, colon cancer is the one which is most characteristic of modern Western culture," Burkitt said. "Colorectal cancer is always rare amongst primitive people. It is nonexistent in undomesticated animals. The only animals that get it are highly domesticated animals like dogs and pigs. Everything points to diet, and the most important things in diet are fat and fiber."

Here, again, fat is a culprit. But, to an extent, fiber helps counteract its effects. After a meal, the gallbladder releases bile acids into the intestine to help absorb the fats we have eaten. Bacteria in the intestine turn these bile acids into cancer-promoting substances called secondary bile acids. And this is where fiber comes in, as Dr. Burkitt points out, "Fiber in the diet alters the bacteria in the intestine and reduces the breakdown of primary into secondary bile acids. In addition, fiber absorbs these bile acids the same way that blotting paper absorbs spilled ink. It gets them out of the way. It also dilutes them into a large stool instead of a small stool. So they are reduced, absorbed, and diluted. So in a nutshell, fat would seem to be promotive, and fiber would be protective."

Bile acids are normal. We need them to absorb fat and for other digestive functions. But when these bile acids change into cancer-causing secondary bile acids, we need fiber to minimize this process and to get them out of the way.

Just as colon cancer is rare in countries with a high-fiber diet, a similar pattern is evident with breast cancer. In part, this is because a diet that is high in fiber tends to be low in fat, and a low-fat diet helps reduce risk of breast cancer. But the story is more complex than that. Fiber, it appears, actually offers additional protection.

"There's some evidence suggesting that fiber may be protective against breast cancer," Burkitt said. Again, changes in sex hormones may be responsible. But it is not only dietary fat which changes them; fiber affects hormones as well. "The risk of breast cancer is directly related to the age of menarche, the age when girls reach puberty. In America in the middle of the last century, puberty started at seventeen. Now it's thirteen. In an African village it will be seventeen; in Johannesburg it will be thirteen. A group in Wales under a man called Hughes looked at 46 countries to see what he could find related to age of menarche, and the only thing that related to age of menarche was fiber intake. Fiber affects cholesterol metabolism, and cholesterol is a precursor of the hormones that regulate uterine growth."

By increasing fiber intake, cholesterol levels are reduced. The theory, then, is that reducing cholesterol, in turn, may reduce the levels of hormones which lead to cancer. A second mechanism comes from the fact that waste estrogens are excreted into the intestine via the bile ducts, along with the digestive juices. Fiber helps carry them away. If there is not much fiber in the diet, these waste estrogens can be reabsorbed back into the bloodstream. Of course, increasing fiber intake generally also means decreasing fat intake. In any case, the result is less breast cancer. For now, these are theories, but they help explain the dramatically different ages of sexual maturity and the marked differences in breast cancer rates in groups with different diets.

"Breast cancer is also related to a longer period elapsing between the onset of puberty and the first full-term pregnancy," Burkitt said. "Now if you have a late menarche, then you don't have a long time between menarche and first pregnancy." And your cancer risk is reduced.

If a low-fat, high-fiber diet actually raises the age of puberty to a more appropriate age, one might wonder what effect it might have on social problems such as teenage pregnancy. But the bottom line is that diet is likely to be very important in breast cancer risk.

Where can modern Westerners find rich sources of fiber? Whole wheat bread, cereals, brown rice, and other whole grains retain the fiber that is lost from refined grains. Beans and vegetables are also rich in fiber. Fiber is only found in plants; no foods from animal sources contain fiber. In Chapter 6, Dr. Burkitt tells us much more about the value of fiber in preventing common illnesses.

Protein and Protein Sources

There is also evidence linking a high intake of protein, particularly animal protein, to some types of cancer. In part, this is because foods that are high in protein, such as beef, are often high in fat and lacking in fiber as well. But it appears that excess protein itself may increase cancer risk. The National Research Council stated, " . . . evidence from both epidemiological and laboratory studies suggests that high protein intake may be associated with an increased risk of cancers at certain sites."[2] The international study of Armstrong and Doll implicated meat and animal protein in several cancers. Diets that are too high in protein have been linked to cancers of the breast, colon, rectum, pancreas, uterus, and prostate.[3]

Research has implicated animal proteins more than other sources of protein. One reason may be the tendency of chemicals such as DDT to concentrate in animal tissues. DDT is still commonly found in meats, years after it was banned. Is this a serious problem in terms of cancer risk?

"It's a very reasonable question," Alabaster said. "I don't think we have the evidence one way or another at the moment. But certainly if you're trying to minimize your risk, you're going to identify risk factors, some of which may be well-established, while others are theoretical. As Immanuel Kant said, 'It is often necessary to make a decision on the basis of knowledge sufficient for action but insufficient to satisfy the intellect.' I think we have to act on our best information. Put the question the other way around: If you know that animal food sources contain a lot of these substances which you know are potentially harmful, it doesn't make a whole lot of sense to go on eating them."

> *"If you know that animal food sources contain a lot of these substances which you know are potentially harmful, it doesn't make a whole lot of sense to go on eating them."*
>
> **Dr. Oliver Alabaster**

The fat content of our meals should be no more than one-half to one-fourth of current amounts. Our protein intake should be scaled back as well. Together, these will help protect against cancer. But there is much more we can do.

Dairy Products and Cancer

There is preliminary evidence that dairy products may contribute to cancer of the ovary, which occurs in 1.5 percent of American women. The culprit is actually a breakdown product of the milk sugar *lactose*. Lactose is broken down in the body to form another sugar called *galactose*, which, in turn, is broken down further by a group of enzymes. According to a study by Dr. Daniel Cramer and his colleagues at Harvard, when dairy product consumption exceeds the enzymes' capacity to break down galactose, there is a build-up of galactose in the blood, which may affect a woman's ovaries.[9] Some women have particularly low levels of a certain enzyme and can only break down galactose very slowly. When they consume dairy products on a regular basis, their risk of ovarian cancer can be triple that of other women. Since the problem is the milk sugar, rather than milk fat, it is not solved by using non-fat products. In fact, yogurt and cottage cheese seem to be of most concern because the bacteria used in their production increase the production of galactose from lactose. People who have no problem with the lactose sugar may still have difficulty metabolizing galactose.

There are other reasons to suspect that galactose can damage the ovary. People who consume more dairy products and have a greater tendency to make galactose from lactose actually have higher rates of infertility. This is particularly true for those in the later child-bearing years. The reason, apparently, is ovarian damage.[10]

What Cramer found was an association between dairy products and ovarian cancer, and a logical explanation to back it up. Further studies of people with ovarian cancer are needed for confirmation of this link. But it is, nonetheless, an important issue, because dairy product consumption is very widespread, yet quite new from an evolutionary standpoint. Before about 4,000 B.C., there was no dairy product consumption by anyone except for the milk consumed by breast-feeding infants. It is apparent that there are some toxicities to humans from the consumption of cows' milk. Although some of these are relatively mild, such as allergies and lactose intolerance, others may be more serious.

Vitamins, Minerals, and Free Radicals

Micronutrients are parts of the diet that are required in only very small amounts: vitamins, minerals, and trace elements. They just might be the David that can slay the Goliath of cancer. To see how they work, we need to take a look at how cancer develops.

As a normal part of body chemistry, molecules called *free radicals* are produced, which can damage the DNA in our cells. Evidence suggests that this damage may lead to cancer. Compounds which block the effects of free radicals may help prevent cancer. "Free radicals are like a terrorist group that tours around creating havoc," Alabaster said. "They are highly unstable molecules. The hypothesis is that in their search for stability, they actually end up attacking cellular DNA. They may damage the DNA in such a way that the cell is transformed into a cancer cell."

Damage from free radicals is also implicated in the aging process and heart disease. Fats, especially polyunsaturated ones, enhance free radical production. Alabaster points out, "Saturated fats are bad for heart disease but may be slightly less harmful from the point of view of cancer risk. Conversely, polyunsaturated fats are better for heart disease and perhaps slightly worse for cancer risk But the difference is not profound. Of course, if one is dropping the fat intake from 45 percent to 20 percent, you're so drastically reducing all types of fat that one hopes that any subtle differences between different types of fat would be essentially negated."

Happily, there are foods which can neutralize the free radicals which have formed. These are called antioxidants. Beta-carotene, vitamins C and E, and the mineral selenium all have antioxidant properties. These compounds can neutralize free radicals and potentially limit the damage that contributes to cancer and possibly to aging and heart disease as well.

Beta-carotene occurs naturally in dark green, yellow, and orange vegetables. In the body, beta-carotene becomes vitamin A. Researchers at the National Cancer Institute are finding that beta-carotene and vitamin A help protect against cancer. For example, asbestos workers, particularly those who smoke, are at tremendous risk for lung cancer. But they are protected somewhat when their diet includes foods rich in beta-carotene.

"Up until now," says NCI's Peter Greenwald, "we really haven't been able to do anything for those people except to tell them not to smoke. We don't have a good means of early detection for lung cancer. So the study aims to see if we can prevent the onset of cancer." Studies of this type showed significant benefits from beta-carotene and vitamin A. "There are over twenty epidemiological studies," Greenwald said. "These studies show that populations having diets high in beta-carotene or vitamin A have lower cancer rates. I do want to emphasize that smokers still would be at a tremendously high risk of lung cancer, and they should stop smoking. They should not hold their breath in the hope that beta-carotene or vitamin A will prevent lung cancer, even if it somewhat lowers risk. People should not feel they're safe from cancer if they take a vitamin pill."

Vitamin A supplements are not generally recommended, as it can be quite toxic in overdose. The amounts of beta-carotene in foods supply a safe and helpful amount of vitamin A. Carrots, broccoli, spinach, apricots, asparagus, kale, cantaloupe, mangoes, peaches, sweet potatoes, and many other vegetables are rich in beta-carotene.

Vitamin C is also an antioxidant with the potential to help prevent cancer. Citrus fruits are well-known for their vitamin C content, but many vegetables are rich sources too; broccoli, Brussels sprouts, asparagus, cauliflower, cabbage, sweet potatoes, tomatoes, and other vegetables contain vitamin C. Some cancer researchers also advocate taking supplementary vitamin C, on the order of about 1000 milligrams per day.

> *"Smokers should not hold their breath in the hope that beta-carotene or vitamin A will prevent lung cancer, even if it somewhat lowers risk. People should not feel they're safe from cancer if they take a vitamin pill."*
>
> **Dr. Peter Greenwald**

Vitamin E, like vitamins A and C, is an antioxidant, protecting against the genetic damage which may lead to cancer. Vitamin E is found in grains and vegetable oils.

Selenium is a mineral which also promotes antioxidant activity and may help prevent cancer. Whole grains are a good source of selenium, although their selenium content varies from one geographic location to another. Caution is advised regarding supplements; selenium is toxic in large amounts. Animal sources of selenium, such as liver and kidney, are not recommended because of their high content of fat and cholesterol.

If your diet includes a generous amount of whole grain cereals or breads, a variety of dark green and yellow vegetables, beans, and fruits, you will be tapping the best sources of beta-carotene, vitamins C and E, and selenium. In addition, these foods contribute fiber, which is also very important.

In spite of our best efforts, free radicals will do some DNA damage. Fortunately, the body has another line of defense. It can actually repair damaged DNA. To do so, it needs folic acid, a B vitamin found in dark green leafy vegetables, fruits, wheat germ, dried peas and beans, and other foods. Human experiments have shown that folic acid helps repair chromosomal damage, as Alabaster relates. "Folic acid has been found in human experiments to protect cells against damage by powerful mutagens, such as caffeine. A mutagen like caffeine causes breaks at fragile sites in chromosomes. The fragile sites that are susceptible to mutagens are also the sites that have been found to be damaged in virtually all human solid tumors. If you take human volunteers and load them up with a high dose of folic acid and then give them the mutagen, you get no damage to the chromosomes. The implication of this work is that a diet rich in folic acid should optimize your DNA repair pathways, limiting the damage of carcinogens.

"So if you used antioxidants to inhibit free radical damage in the first place and folic acid to enhance repair in the second place," Alabaster said, "you may end up with more stable cells."

There are other cancer-fighting micronutrients as well. Cruciferous vegetables, that is, broccoli, cauliflower, Brussels sprouts, and cabbage contain natural chemicals called *indoles* and *aromatic isothiocyanates*, which help prevent cancer. Garlic and onions contain large quantities of *quercetin*, a natural chemical which appears to have anti-cancer properties. In China, people who consume large quantities of garlic and onions (about three ounces a day) have less than half the risk of stomach cancer compared to those who consume only an ounce per day of these vegetables. And Alabaster mentions several other naturally occurring substances which may have cancer-fighting properties.

"Phenols occur naturally in many vegetables and artificially as the preservative BHA. Flavones are found in many fruits and vegetables. Protease inhibitors are also anticarcinogens, and they are found in soybeans, various seeds, and lima beans. Beta-sitosterol is also found in many vegetables and vegetable oils. Another is glutathione, which is present in many of our foods and which has been found to have anticarcinogenic and antioxidant properties and therefore can be very protective."

In addition, many foods contain *antimutagens* which may help prevent cancer. A mutagen is a substance which damages the cells' DNA. This damage may lead to cancer. Antimutagens help protect the cells. "Many foods contain antimutagenic properties," Alabaster said. "Extracts from broccoli, cabbage, green pepper, eggplant, shallots, pineapple, apples, ginger, and mint leaf have all been shown to have antimutagenic activity, without necessarily identifying which

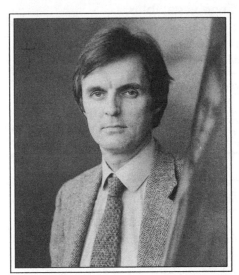

Dr. Oliver Alabaster

components of these extracts are the active ingredients. Wheat sprouts, parsley, lettuce, Brussels sprouts, spinach, mustard greens, and other vegetables have also been found to be antimutagenic. Lettuce contains anti-mutagens, but also contains carcinogenic activity as well."

So there are some confusing areas here. Some foods have combinations of effects. Some of their components may help fight cancer, while other components of the same food may *cause* cancer. The question, then, is what is the dominant property of each food.

What are the best bets? Vegetables are essential. Dark green and yellow vegetables supply beta-carotene and vitamin C. The cruciferous vegetables contribute indoles and isothyocyanates. Whole grains in cereals and breads contribute vitamin E and selenium. And vegetables, fruits, grains, and beans supply fiber and are naturally low in fat.

Food Constituents That May Help Prevent Cancer

ELEMENTS	SOURCES
fiber	grains, beans, vegetables, fruits
beta-carotene	dark green, yellow, and orange vegetables, *(such as carrots, broccoli, spinach, apricots, asparagus, kale, cantaloupe, mangoes, peaches, sweet potatoes)*
vitamin C	broccoli, Brussels sprouts, asparagus, cauliflower, cabbage, sweet potatoes, tomatoes, citrus fruits
vitamin E	whole grains
selenium	whole grains
indoles, isothiocyanates	cruciferous vegetables: *(Brussels sprouts, cabbage, cauliflower, and broccoli)*

A New Dietary Balance

Alabaster, Burkitt, Greenwald, and Bailar each have their own ideas on eating to prevent cancer. From my own perspective, an optimal diet for cancer prevention means eliminating meats and dairy products, which are always devoid of fiber and frequently much too high in fat and protein. It means avoiding fried foods and added oils. And it means having generous amounts of whole grains, legumes, fruits, and vegetables. Any shift toward this optimal diet is a shift toward health.

"The fact that chemical pollution is responsible for a relatively small percentage of cancer cases and diet and smoking are responsible for 70-80 percent suggests that the bulk of cancer can be modified by decisions we make ourselves," Alabaster said. "We don't have to wait for the federal government to do something. We can actually do something right now. The basic message that should be conveyed is that at least 70 percent of cancer is thought to be preventable based on what we now know. That is an astonishing figure which I would never have guessed at five years ago."

What we can do then is to stack the odds very much in our favor by cutting our fat intake, doubling our fiber intake, and including in our diet the cancer-fighting vitamins and minerals found naturally in plants.

While research continues, NCI's Greenwald feels that we know enough to change our diet. "What we recommend is a variety of foods that are high in fiber, low in fat, and keeping trim." Our meal plans should favor "fresh or frozen vegetables, fruits, and whole grain cereals and breads."

> *"The fact that chemical pollution is responsible for a relatively small percentage of cancer cases and diet and smoking are responsible for 70-80 percent suggests that the bulk of cancer can be modified by decisions we make ourselves."*
>
> **Dr. Oliver Alabaster**

Steps To Cancer Prevention

- ◆ Do not use tobacco in any form.
- ◆ Avoid fried foods and added oils.
- ◆ Increase fiber to about 40 grams daily by including more whole grains, beans, and vegetables in the diet.

- ◆ Eliminate foods from animal sources. Vegetarian diets are linked to the lowest cancer rates.

- ◆ Increase intake of dark green, orange and yellow vegetables. Also, make the cruciferous vegetables, such as broccoli, Brussels sprouts, cabbage, and cauliflower, a regular part of the diet.

- ◆ Limit alcohol intake to no more than one drink per day or the equivalent.

- ◆ Maintain your weight at or near your ideal weight.

- ◆ Avoid exposure to excessive sunlight or unnecessary X-rays.

Changing Medicine, Changing Ourselves

Doctors, like people in general, are slow to change. We don't alter old habits or outlooks without a struggle. John Bailar's revelations in the *New England Journal of Medicine* of May 8, 1986, that we are making little progress with cancer treatment and need a radically different approach was met with defensiveness by some cancer researchers.

"There is a degree of momentum in any big program that can be a very powerful force," Bailar said. "A change at NCI of the kind I'm describing, from perhaps three-to-one support for treatment over prevention to a one-to-two ratio the other way, would mean a massive disruption in ideas, in momentum, in the research community, in the businesses that support that research community. Mainly it means a massive disruption in the way people have been thinking for decades, and this is very difficult to do. I recognize that, particularly where you have a large organization that has a substantial planning effort and feels it has done good research management for a long period of time. Such people don't take kindly to criticism."

Perhaps there is a psychological reason, as well. In my medical school class, there was one fellow who always wore his surgical garb wherever he was, whether he was in the operating room or not. He dreamed of being a medical hero, a

Ben Casey. Unfortunately, he would practice medicine the way another famous Casey played baseball. The cocky athlete let the first and then the second pitch go by without bothering to swing. He let the tension build toward the dramatic home run he would hit at the last possible moment. But when the final pitch flew, his bat missed it completely. He struck out.

> *"Prevention is going to be a lot less dramatic than treatment and cure. You can point to individual victims of cancer. You'll never be able to point to people who have been saved from cancer by prevention."*
>
> **Dr. John Bailar**

As Bailar points out, "Certainly, prevention is going to be a lot less dramatic than treatment and cure. You can point to individual victims of cancer. You'll never be able to point to people who have been saved from cancer by prevention."

In the fight against cancer, we let our chance to prevent illness fly by, hoping to be able to cure disease when it develops. We fight cancer only when it is big enough to feel with our hands or see on an X-ray. At that point, our batting average is very poor indeed. In the process, our patients, our spouses, our children, and ourselves are at tremendous risk.

NCI had set as its explicit goal to reduce cancer deaths by fifty percent by the year 2000. Still, that goal is nowhere in sight. Cancer deaths continue to climb. Winning the War on Cancer will require a redirection of our research efforts toward a new emphasis on prevention.

"It's very hard to make anybody take a risk seriously which expresses itself over a 20-year period," Alabaster said. "They live for the day, the week, or the month at the very most. It's extremely hard to make people plan ahead. Changing dietary habits requires people to be willing to take steps now to reduce their risk of something years ahead. It takes a whole insurance industry to sell life insurance policies and retirement plans. And they promise financial return in the short run as well as the benefits to the family in the long run. We don't have an equivalent army selling cancer prevention. If we had thousands of agents, as it were, pestering everybody, maybe we'd get somewhere. Of course, the real agents ought to be medical professionals. It requires physicians to realize that they have a responsibility to try to prevent disease as well as to treat it, something which is usually underemphasized in medical education.

"Preventive measures are really the way of the future. They have also been the way of the past. A hundred years ago, half the population was dead before the age of forty, mainly because of infection. Now that number is down to three percent, due to preventive measures: better sanitation, better hygiene, vaccinations, and to a very small extent direct therapy. This is a dramatic change produced by preventive measures. The three major killer diseases that now account for premature mortality are cancer, heart disease, and stroke. They account for four out of five deaths. Yet these three diseases are largely untreatable and almost entirely preventable if we make the right decisions. So the three major killer diseases which will otherwise be with us well into the next century could be nearly abolished if we take the right steps."

> *"It requires physicians to realize that they have a responsibility to try to prevent disease as well as to treat it, something which is usually underemphasized in medical education."*
>
> **Dr. Oliver Alabaster**

The key, then is to return not only to the time-tested methods of prevention, but to the time-tested eating habits of the past. "Our modern diet is really an anathema to our whole historical evolution," Alabaster said. "Why should we expect our bodies to react well to it? In the evolutionary time scale, meat is a relatively new phenomenon. It used to be that fruit, nuts, cereal, and vegetation were really the basis of the human diet over the millennia. The good news is that we now realize that we can, to a great degree, control our risks of cancer and other diseases through decisions we make ourselves. I hope we will take advantage of it."

Chapter 4

New Strategies for Weight Control

There is a new approach to weight control which is far more effective in maintaining permanent results than any "diet."

This chapter presents a strategy that works. With this plan, you can drop to your best weight. The improvement is permanent—no more ups and downs on the scale. But it is not a "diet" in the sense of going hungry with skimpy portions. You can feel full and satisfied at every meal. Earning these dividends requires an investment: it requires shifting your attention from *how much* you are eating to *what* you are eating. You must also give some attention to timing: when you eat can be as important as what you eat.

First, we will restructure the menu. Certain foods allow you to eat more, if you like, while staying slimmer. Other foods, particularly those that do not help maintain an active metabolism or are packed with dense calories, should be avoided. We will also take a look at physical activity and ways to bring it into your life, and genetic and medical factors. While most overweight people actually eat less than thin people, if you do overeat, we will take a look at what's eating you, and how to deal with it.

In addition, there are ways to burn calories more quickly. You have seen people who never seem to gain weight no matter how much they eat. What they have going for them is a metabolism that rapidly burns off calories. You can adjust your metabolism in two ways: food choices and physical activity. We will look at both.

It is Not *How Much* You Eat; It's *What* You Eat

Many diets rely on restricting the amount of food you eat. This can work only for so long. Soon, the natural desire for food brings weight back up to where you started—and often beyond—because the diet has caused a slowing of the metabolism, making every calorie harder to burn off. Of course, those who really are stuffing themselves do need to cut back, but the vast majority of overweight people will lose weight by simply changing food choices.

Studies have shown that most overweight people do not eat more than thin people. Let us take a look, not at *how much* you eat, but at *what* to eat.

Fat In Foods Is Fat On You

Fats are the most calorie-dense parts of the foods we eat. Every gram of fat or oil holds nine calories. This is true for all fats and oils: beef fat, chicken fat, fish oil, or vegetable oil. In contrast, carbohydrates, such as the inside of a potato, or beans, rice, or pasta, have only four calories per gram, less than half the calories than the same amount of fat.

An average American consumes nearly half his calories, about 40 percent, as fat. For a person eating 2,000 calories per day, that is 800 calories each day just from fats and oils in our foods.

Think about animal fat. Animal fat was the calorie-storage area of the animal it came from. So when you eat animal fat, you are eating all those stored calories. My uncle was a cattle rancher. I remember riding with him to East St. Louis to sell a load of cattle. He used to tell me with pride about how the fat was "marbled" throughout the meat to make it juicier. Although people may trim the white strip off the edge of a cut of meat, people like my uncle make sure that meats are permeated with fat, like a sponge holding water.

Fat in foods finds its way very easily into our body fat. Little or no conversion is needed in the body before the fat we eat is added to the fat tissues of the body. So don't eat someone else's fat. It will put fat on you.

William Connor is a well-known researcher in the field of nutrition and health. With his wife Sonja, he wrote *The New American Diet,* (Simon & Schuster, 1986) and is a frequent lecturer at medical conferences. He became concerned about the dangers of a high-fat diet while he was a resident at the University of Iowa Hospital.

"I had a patient I was very fond of who had very high blood fat levels. While we were in the course of doing some studies to evaluate him, he dropped dead suddenly while playing cards. This was before the days of cardiac resuscitation. Outside of injecting adrenaline into his chest, there was not much we could do. There wasn't CPR. He had an autopsy and I looked at the coronary arteries. They were clogged with fat. I became convinced that this was an important area to study and that nutrition would affect all these factors a great deal."

Connor is concerned about the amount of fat Americans are eating. "My wife Sonja has a very good demonstration that she calls 'the fats of life.' She shows how much fat is in a cheeseburger, that is, how many pats of butter it would take to have as much fat as is in the cheeseburger—in the cheese, in the mayonnaise, and in the meat. It turns out to be a fabulous number, about 13 pats of butter, which she puts out on a plate. No one can contemplate directly eating 13 pats of butter, but they essentially do when they eat a cheeseburger."

> *"No one can contemplate directly eating 13 pats of butter, but they essentially do when they eat a cheeseburger."*
>
> **Dr. William Connor**

Let's take another example: imagine that we're making tacos. We have two recipes for taco filling, one made with ground beef, which is a high-fat food, and the other from beans, which are very low in fat. Three ounces of ground beef contains about 225 calories, but the same amount of beans has only about 80 calories. The difference is the very low fat content of beans.

You have probably been told that lean beef, chicken, and fish are low-fat foods. This is poor advice, as you know if you have tried to lose weight by eating them. These foods are low in fat only in comparison to the worst foods, such as beef or pork. Poultry, fish, and all meats contain significant amounts of inherent fat. A 3½ oz. piece of roasted chicken holds about 240 calories, a large portion of which is fat. If you strip off the skin and throw away the dark meat, you are still left with plenty of calories, about 173 (the chicken also contributes about 85 mg. of cholesterol).[1] Contrast that with a baked potato weighing the same amount, holding only 95 calories. The potato contains carbohydrate, protein, vitamins, and minerals, but very little fat. So it is naturally low in calories. Chicken, like all meats, is permeated by fat and has no carbohydrate or fiber. Likewise fish oils, like all fats and oils, contain nine calories per gram.

Animal fats are not the only offenders. Vegetable oils are packed with calories too. For example, a baked potato contains about 95 calories and virtually no fat. If the same potato were turned into french fries, it would contain more than 270 calories, because of all the oil used in frying. Nuts and seeds are also high in vegetable oil and high in calories. It's no good eliminating meats if you are just going to substitute oil-rich french fries and onion rings. The key is to minimize fats and oils from whatever source, because, again, any fat or oil contains nine calories per gram, compared to only four for carbohydrate or protein.

You may be saying that you hardly eat any fat. Ask yourself if you eat meat, poultry, fish, cheese, nuts, or fried foods. If so, you are eating much more fat than you realize, because these foods all have inherent fat. That extra bit of fat is displacing the carbohydrate and fiber that you need.

To compare the leanest meats to a meat-free menu, let us imagine three different meals. One dinner is a typical vegetarian dinner of black beans, white rice, and broccoli spears. Black beans are among the most savory varieties of beans, and

quite prominent in the cooking of Mexico's Yucatan peninsula and other Latin American countries. Let us compare that
meal to a dinner that is the same in all respects except that
instead of beans we will have lean beef, and to another meal
which will include skinless roast chicken breast instead of
beans. These are about as lean as beef and chicken can get. But
even though the lean beef and chicken meals are lower in fat
than other meat meals, they contain significantly more fat,
more calories, and less fiber and carbohydrate than the vegetarian dinner. Table 1 shows the difference meals of this type
can make over the course of seven days.

Table 1. Vegetarian Dinner vs. Lean Meat Dinners
A Comparison of a Week's Worth of Nutrients

	Beans, rice, and broccoli	Chicken, rice, and broccoli	Lean beef, rice and broccoli
Fat (g)	3.5	34.3	51.1
Calories (kcal)	1,790	2,180	2,480
Protein (g)	88	252	288
Carbohydrate	365	278	208
Fiber	40	15	15

This table compares seven days of each of three dinners.
The meals were a typical vegetarian dinner including 4 oz. of
black beans, a typical lean beef meal including 4 oz. of lean
top round roast, and a meal including 4 oz. of roast chicken
breast with no skin. All dinners also included ½ cup of white
rice and ½ cup of broccoli.

As the table shows, even the "leanest" beef and chicken
contain far more fat than the vegetarian meal. Even though
only white chicken meat was used and the skin was removed,
the chicken meal still adds more than 30 extra grams of fat and
almost 400 extra calories every week, compared to the same
size serving of beans. The lean beef adds nearly 50 extra grams
of fat in a week. And because chicken and all other meats

contain no fiber and no carbohydrate, there are obvious differences in both. Seven days of either the chicken or beef meals contains about 600 mg. of cholesterol, which you definitely do not need. The chicken also contains a large quantity of protein, far more than the body needs. This extra protein simply contributes more calories and other adverse health consequences that we will review in Chapter 6.

If this same eating pattern also holds for breakfast and lunch, you can see the price you pay when you include even modest amounts of "lean" meats in your regular menu. Over the long run, they add calories, while displacing fiber and carbohydrate. So you feel less satisfied after meals, have less of the calorie-burning effect of carbohydrate (see +), and get a regular dose of calorie-rich fat. Note that this example used "lean" meats. Most diets which include meat are even worse, because they are much higher in fat, and, of course, contain no carbohydrate or fiber at all. This is not to say that lean meats are not healthier than fatty meats; they are. But they have nowhere near the power of low-fat vegetarian meals to promote permanent weight control.

The human body does need some fat in the diet. But the amount we need is only a fraction of what most of us typically get. A certain modest amount of fat is inherent in grains and vegetables. This is all the body needs. The only exception would be for small children: breast milk contains fat for the needs of growing infants. The natural process of weaning eliminates this nutrient when it is no longer appropriate. In early childhood, a bit more fat than adults should have may be allowed in the diet.

In practical terms, the most potent weight-control diet includes plenty of grains, such as breads, rice, and pasta, as well as beans, vegetables, and fruits. It excludes meats, poultry, fish, high-fat dairy products, fried foods, and added oil. Getting away from fats is a great feeling. Enjoy eating generous portions of spaghetti with tomato sauce, vegetable curries and bean burritos, with delicious breads and vegetables. Enjoy the natural taste of vegetables or salads without oily dressings or with some of the delicious new low-fat or non-fat dressings now out on the market.

You will find that you can rapidly adapt to a new way of eating. It does take an adjustment though, because people crave high-calorie foods, unfortunately. Fats and oils attract us like addicting substances. This manifests in the form of binges on fried chicken, greasy burgers, potato chips, or chocolate. It may be that an inherent attraction to high-calorie foods helped our species to avoid starvation. During famines of the past, those who knew a good source of calories when they saw one survived. Those who did not avail themselves of calorie-rich foods might have starved. So if you look like you are wearing a total-body life-preserver, maybe you are. It's just that you don't need it anymore.

It helps to remember that fatty foods act like addicting substances. You will have a tendency to return to them, so be on the look-out. I suggest cutting them out almost entirely so that you are not continually teasing yourself and maintaining the taste for these foods. The modest amounts of naturally occurring oils in grains and vegetables will prevent a deficiency of any fats the body needs.

Carbohydrates: Naturally Low in Calories

Many diet books have charts of the calorie content of foods and tell you how much (or how little) you have to eat to lose weight. They indicate that all foods are equivalent as long as they contain the same number of calories. But it turns out that calories from carbohydrates are not as likely to increase body fat as is the same number of calories from fats. Why this is so is not entirely clear, but there are some clues: the body has to do a fair amount of work to store the energy of carbohydrates. The process of converting carbohydrates to fat consumes some calories. In contrast, the body finds it quite easy to add the fat in foods to the fat already stored on your abdomen, your thighs, or other fat storage areas. Much less conversion is needed.

You may be thinking that carbohydrates are fattening. If you have been avoiding carbohydrate-rich potatoes, rice, and pasta because you thought they were fattening, stop worrying. They are, in fact, low-calorie foods. It is only when starches are covered in fatty toppings that lots of calories are added. For example, spaghetti is modest in calories. But when it is topped with a greasy ground beef sauce, the calories are packed in. Or when potatoes are topped with butter or sour cream, a low-calorie food becomes a high-calorie food. In other words, *fatty toppings* are high in calories, but the carbohydrates themselves are not. An ounce of carbohydrate has *less than half the calories of an ounce of fat.*

Concentrated sugars are one form of carbohydrate that does contain more calories than we need, and dieters have for years blamed sugars for their problems. To an extent this is justified. Sugars are as concentrated a form of calories as can be found in a carbohydrate food. But even so, sugars are not nearly as calorie-dense as fats. If you are not controlling

> *"Sugars are not nearly as calorie-dense as fats. If you are not controlling the amount of fat you are eating, there is little point in worrying about sugar."*
>
> **Dr. Neal Barnard**

the amount of fat you are eating, there is little point in worrying about sugar. Sugar is also better than the artificial flavoring NutraSweet. There is no convincing evidence that this chemical helps control weight, and it is implicated in convulsions and other nervous system problems. As we will see in Chapter 7, children and pregnant women are strongly advised to avoid it, and that is good advice for everyone else as well.

A word about alcohol: all forms of alcohol contain plenty of calories. A bottled beer contains about 150 calories. Four ounces of wine or champagne contain about 85 calories. Alcohol is a source of extra calories which tends to add the pounds, in addition to the many other serious problems that can be caused by excessive alcohol use. [2,3]

Fiber: The Added Dividend In Plants

For a long time, all that doctors knew about fiber was that polyester suits were cheap. But we have come a long way. By now, everyone has heard of fiber's value in maintaining health. Fiber also helps keep weight under control. As a natural part of foods, fiber gives them a hearty, satisfying texture but has virtually no calories.

What is fiber? It is what people used to call roughage—the part of plants that resists digestion in the small intestine. Unfortunately, the refining methods used in recent decades have taken the fiber out of foods, so that breads, baked goods, and cereals are more densely packed with calories and less satisfying. Happily, that is starting to change. More and more food producers are leaving the fiber in some of their products. Brown rice, whole wheat bread, whole grain cereals, and pastas are making their comeback. These foods are both satisfying and naturally low in calories.

Grains (such as wheat, oats, rice, and the breads, cereals, and other foods that are made from them), beans, lentils, and other legumes, and many vegetables are rich in carbohydrate and fiber, while still very low in fat. Fiber comes only from plants. Foods from animal sources contain no fiber at all.

Don't Overdo It with Protein

The best advice about protein is to forget it. Most plants contain at least ten percent protein. So even without meats, your foods will contain plenty of protein, and you need not go out of your way to get more of it. High-protein diets, in fact, are harmful.

Some weight-loss diets, such as the approach in Dr. Robert Atkins' *Diet Revolution* (Bantam, 1972), are very high in protein and contain very little carbohydrate. While this can result in a rapid water loss, it is not a long-term solution to overweight. The reason is this: the body needs sugar in the blood stream in order to function. The sugar normally comes from carbohydrate. If there is no carbohydrate in the diet, the body breaks down protein to manufacture sugar.

C. Wayne Callaway, M.D., is a well-known medical consultant to nutrition journals and has served on the faculties of the Mayo Clinic and the George Washington University School of Medicine. He believes that high-protein, low-carbohydrate diets are dangerous. "If you're not taking in carbohydrate, you will break down protein," Callaway said. "When that happens, for every ounce of protein you break down, there are three ounces of water that are released, because that water has been surrounding the protein molecule."

That water is then lost, so water weight comes off tempo-
rarily. But you cannot keep this up for long. Soon, the water
and weight will come back on. And there are dangers as well.
Too much protein in the diet contributes to osteoporosis, as
we will see in Chapter 6. In addition, it forces the kidneys to
overwork. "High-protein diets may accelerate the decline in
kidney function, especially in people who already have some
degree of kidney impairment for whatever reason," Callaway
said. "There's no good reason to recommend more protein."

High-protein diets of any kind are unnecessary and harmful. If you eat a varied diet, you will be getting enough protein,
and it is best not to overdo it. High-protein diets are no
solution to being overweight.

The worst problem with protein is that Americans have
lived in fear of not getting enough. This has led them to
include meats and dairy products in their daily routines, with
predictable consequences: they get fat. There is more than
enough protein in grains, beans, and vegetables, with much
less fat.

International Foods, Vegetarian Foods

Foods that come from plants are generally rich in carbohydrate, moderate in protein, and low in fat. Unfortunately, so
many Western foods are based on animal products. Many
other countries have developed far healthier culinary traditions. They use much smaller amounts of meat than are
typically used in America and other Western nations. Meatless meals are common in the traditional foods of the Middle
East, Asia, Latin America, and Africa. Italian pastas, Mexican
beans, rice, and tortillas, Indian curries, Asian rice and vegetables—provided they are not topped with fatty sauces—are
often excellent choices. While the more well-to-do people in
these countries often adopt a Westernized, meat-based diet
and pay the price in obesity, diabetes, heart disease, and other
problems, those who remain on largely vegetarian, traditional
diets tend to remain slim.

Even in America, this idea is hardly new. A quote from
history: "I have lived temperately, eating little animal food,
and not as an aliment, so much as a condiment for the

vegetables which constitute my principal diet." That was how Thomas Jefferson described his own eating habits, as Dr. Connor relates: "The word 'aliment' means the chief aspect of the meal. In a restaurant, the menu is written in terms of the meat items: fish, chicken, steak. Everything else is distributed in smaller quantities around the meat dish. Jefferson's idea was to use the meat to spice up the carbohydrates, the starches, the vegetables, and so on. So you use a small quantity, like a condiment. If you use pepper you don't use a lot of pepper; you use only a little. Meat should be thought of in the same way."

Connor notes that many other great figures in history have avoided meat and, intentionally or not, avoided the fat, cholesterol, and dense calories of meats in favor of carbohydrates and fiber-rich foods the vegetable kingdom supplies. "If you look at the philosophers and wise people over the ages, many of them are vegetarians. George Bernard Shaw was a vegetarian. Buddha was a vegetarian. I don't know about Jesus, but we presume he probably was too, or ate very little meat."

If we take the best that other countries have to offer, our menu is more varied, more intriguing, and of course, healthier than chicken or beef ever could be.

Burning Calories

All movement burns calories. Whether it is looking at your watch, working around the house, or running a marathon, every bit of movement uses up some calories. The more we move, the more calories we burn. Modern life, unfortunately, has become all too sedentary. Our jobs involve less and less exertion, and, at home, televisions and home computers often fix us in position.

You probably know whether or not you are getting enough physical activity. Most people are not. The natural calorie-burning effect of physical activity has been largely lost by most of us. If that includes you, see how you can build more into your life.

"We recommend having about 2200 calories of energy expenditure over sedentary living each week," Connor says. That means about 300 calories a day over and above sitting or office work. You have to build that into your routine by walking, climbing stairs, and using your muscles whenever you can. It's going to take, on the average, 30-60 minutes a day to do this. Hopefully, you can do it in a constructive way, such as gardening, or sports or recreational activities one might enjoy."

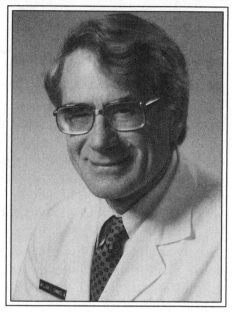

Dr. William Connor

Three hundred calories translates into an hour on the golf course, a half hour jog, or an hour of housework, such as vacuuming. How about dancing? It is terrific exercise. A run with your dog, a vigorous walk in the woods, using the stairs instead of the elevator, a morning or evening walk with a friend—we don't think of these as exercise, but in fact they are great ways to get active. Do you enjoy walking or gardening? How about bike-riding or tennis? Physical movement does not have to be terribly strenuous as long as there is enough of it on a regular basis.

Choose activities that are fun. The "No pain, no gain" philosophy—the idea that there is no profit without suffering—works for some people, but I prefer the "primate approach" to exercise. You may recall films of chimpanzees playing. They wrestle and romp, but when they are tired, they stop. They do not swing from the trees "till it hurts." We don't need to either. We need to learn to play again, as we did when we were children.

Some people enjoy health clubs, which have found creative ways to turn exercise into pleasure. With bright colorful rooms and modern equipment, physical activity can be habit-forming. They have found that many people enjoy exercising on electrical treadmills, rowing machines, or other sophisticated equipment. These inventions provide a fun way to exercise at any speed without getting cold, wet, or windblown.

Physical activity also helps control appetite. Twenty minutes of exercise before dinner helps suppress the appetite for a few hours. There may be a difference between different types of exercise: activities that cool the body, such as swimming may burn more calories as the body tries to restore normal body temperature. But some people experience an *increase* in appetite after cooling exercises. If this is true for you, you may wish to choose a form of exercise that warms the body, such as aerobics or dancing.

If you have been sedentary for some time, it will take a while for your muscles and supporting tissues to tone up. So begin gradually. If you have a history of illness, talk over your plans with your doctor.

The best way to start is with a half-hour walk each day or an hour walk three times per week. It's easy, and it really does help burn the fat.

Turn Up The Flame

Your body is always burning calories. It takes a fair amount of energy just to keep your temperature normal, your brain thinking, dreaming, or even relaxing, your lungs exchanging air, and your heart pumping. Without even lifting a finger, you are always using energy. Your body gets this energy from its stores of fat and various natural sugars in the body. The process of keeping the basic body functions going is referred to as "metabolism." The very slow metabolism of a hibernating bear allows his or her fat to last all winter long without even a scrap of food. If you have been dieting and not losing weight, perhaps your body is "hibernating" in a sense. Your metabolism has slowed in order to conserve the fat you are trying to get rid of.

Many thin people have what is referred to as a "rapid" metabolism. They burn lots of calories in a short period of time. Whether your metabolism is a flicker or a furnace depends on several factors, and *it can be changed*. While your metabolic rate is inherited, to an extent, it can be adjusted up or down somewhat so that the body burns calories faster or slower.

Carbohydrate increases the body's tendency to burn calories.[4-8] "When you digest carbohydrate," Callaway said, "glucose (simple sugar) is released into the blood stream. This causes insulin to be secreted. Insulin does a whole host of things in addition to allowing you to keep your blood sugar normal. Insulin causes a part of the brain, the hypothalamus, to increase the production of norepinephrine. It also probably causes the liver to increase the production of T3, which is the active form of thyroid hormone. T3 and norepinephrine both regulate metabolic rate. When they go up, you burn more calories. So, following a carbohydrate-rich meal there's an increase in your metabolic rate."

Food choices are just one part of the metabolic tune-up. Regular physical activity also alters the metabolism of the body so that it burns calories faster. This is true not only while you are exercising. The effect continues for a period of time, *even while you are at rest.*

There is another way that exercise boosts your metabolism. It builds muscles. Muscle tissue has a rapid metabolism. It burns far more calories than fat tissue does. If we allow our muscles to waste away and we add a bit of fat tissue, we will not burn calories as readily. The meals that would not have caused weight gain previously will now lead to overweight. But the more muscle and less fat we have on our bodies, the more calories we will burn.

No more diets: dieting can slow the metabolism. When you eat less, the body actually tries to conserve fat, so it impedes the body's calorie-burning process. Although this can be very frustrating for dieters, this mechanism evolved long ago when our distant ancestors had to protect themselves from starvation. Just as a motorist who is nearly out of gas tries to conserve fuel until the gas station is in sight, the body of a dieter automatically slows down the metabolism so that not too much fat will be lost before food is once again plentiful. Of course, now we are not trying to conserve our fat stores; we are trying to get rid of them. But our bodies still carry this fat-conserving mechanism. Even worse, the slowed metabolism lasts long beyond the dieting period, so fat is easily and rapidly accumulated again. A study at the University of Pennsylvania showed that very-low-calorie diets can cause a marked slowing of metabolism which persists for several weeks.[9] Even skipping breakfast or lunch on a regular basis can slow the metabolism by about ten percent. The key is to avoid very-low-calorie diets. Weight reduction programs should be gradual, so the metabolism never is slowed.

If you choose to cut back on calories as a temporary measure, be careful. Callaway recommends that, as a rule of thumb, a weight-reduction diet should contain no less than ten calories per pound of body weight.

This, of course, is quite the opposite of what dieters often experience. Their metabolisms have been slowed so severely

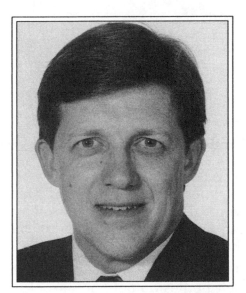

Dr. C. Wayne Callaway

by dieting that even small amounts of food seem to lead to increases on the scale. After a very restrictive diet, an individual can easily gain weight due to fluid retention and because the diet has lowered his or her metabolism. Every calorie eaten is harder to get rid of. They would burn fat better if they had never dieted at all. The solution is to resume a more normal diet with a reasonable number of calories, particularly from starches.

Connor agrees that overly restrictive diets spell long-term failure. "Weight-loss diets should have, for men, 1200-1400 calories or even more, depending on the size of the man, and for women, at least 1000-1200 calories."

If your metabolism has been slowed by a period of low-calorie dieting, increasing your exertion can sometimes make things worse: it can keep your metabolic rate low. Your body is still trying to conserve energy in the face of what it interprets as starvation. So stop the calorie restriction first, then add physical activity.

In summary, the metabolic tune-up is simple: shift your food choices to favor carbohydrates. Cut most fats out of the diet, and have three or four meals during the day, rather than waiting for an evening binge. Then add regular physical activity. You will find that your weight is much easier to control.

Changing Metabolism
- ◆ Increase calorie intake
  (Include no less than 10 calories per pound of body weight in your daily menu)
- ◆ Increase carbohydrates
- ◆ Greatly reduce fatty foods.
- ◆ Regular physical activity

The Restrained-Eater Phenomenon

Binge-eating—it is the worst enemy of the person who wants to slim down. Eating becomes out of control, as if your appetite has taken charge of your life. But we now know why it occurs for many people. And we know how to avoid it. So let's take the mystery out of binging.

Think for a minute about dieters. They stop eating in the hope of losing weight. But their bodies do not know what is going on. The body cannot distinguish dieting from starvation. The human body took shape millions of years ago, when the lack of food meant only one thing: famine. When you stop eating today, your body still interprets skimpy eating as starvation. The body then gets ready to take maximal advantage of any food source it finds. If food then becomes suddenly available, the body reacts as if it has received a temporary food source in the midst of famine. We are automatically driven to gorge ourselves in anticipation of recurrent famine, in what is known as the "restrained eater" phenomenon. Dieters are set-ups for the restrained eater phenomenon.

"If people are undereating, they are frequently not hungry until they start to eat," Callaway said. "When they start to eat, their appetite goes up. Food becomes sort of an appetizer.

"There was an interesting study in which college women were asked to taste different kinds of ice cream. They were under the impression this was some type of taste test or consumer panel. What was really being measured was how much ice cream they were eating. The bowls were on hidden scales. Before they were given the ice cream they had to drink either a milk shake or two milk shakes or nothing. What was found was that the normal eaters did what you would predict. If they had had a milk shake, they ate less ice cream, and after two milk shakes, they ate even less. But the people who were dieting, the "restrained eaters," if they had had a milk shake before they ate, they would eat more ice cream than they did on an empty stomach. If they had had two milk shakes, they'd eat even more."

> *"If people are under-eating, they are frequently not hungry until they start to eat. When they start to eat, their appetite goes up. Food becomes sort of an appetizer."*
>
> **Dr. C. Wayne Callaway**

For the dieters, when food became available, a binge started. A similar effect can even occur in the course of a day, when people skip breakfast and eat a light lunch. After a day of semi-starvation, overeating is likely at dinner.

"The way to avoid that is to eat three meals a day and eat at least the equivalent of what you'd be burning at rest, so you are not chronically starving," Callaway said. "Make sure you have an adequate breakfast," Callaway says. "Twenty to thirty percent of your calories should be breakfast. Lunch should be about thirty to thirty-five percent."

As meals become regularized, your appetite will be much more reasonable as well.

Dieting, Bulimia, and Anorexia Nervosa

For some, the diet-binge cycle gets out of control. It leads to bulimia, in which binging can be followed by self-induced vomiting. Laxatives are sometimes used as well. Secrecy, shame, and a negative self-concept become routine. And the more they try to starve, the more likely they are to binge. The more they binge, the more ashamed they feel. It comes to feel like a moral battle, when in reality, it is a set of predictable biological events that could happen to any dieter.

"It's a very uncomfortable feeling to be out of control, to have that sense of compulsion, becoming more and more hungry as you eat," Callaway said. "This is associated with all kinds of feelings of guilt and secrecy and shame, which you certainly see in young people who have eating disorders. The more they try to starve, the more likely they are to binge. The more they binge, the more likely they are to have further psychological consequences of it."

A tendency to binge can happen to anyone who has been on an overly restrictive diet. There is no reason for shame. But there is every reason to be on a more regular pattern of eating.

The binge-eating of bulimia almost always begins with a diet. The cycle of restrictive dieting and binging would never need to occur if dieting were replaced with reasonable food choices.

In the extreme weight loss of anorexia nervosa, the very low number of calories consumed leads to amenorrhea, that is, the loss of menstrual periods. The victim feels physically and emotionally out of sorts.

"When people starve, their metabolic rate goes down and they end up feeling cold and tired and depressed," Callaway said. "They have dry skin and dry hair. Their blood pressure goes down, so when they stand up they get dizzy and may actually pass out. They almost always get constipated. The mechanical contractions of the stomach and small bowel become very irregular, and they may get cramps, gas, and bloating. They may have diarrhea alternating with constipation."

In serious eating disorders, a combined approach of psychiatric therapy and medical evaluation and information is necessary. The idea of strict dieting should be abandoned in favor of food choices that one can live with permanently. Unfortunately, American teenagers are preoccupied with looking thin. While some attribute this entirely to the fashion industry's preoccupation with thinness, it may also be due to the fact that children are raised on a menu that is almost certain to make many of them gain weight. The cultural trend in Western countries in the past several decades has emphasized meat and dairy products as staples at every meal. Most of these foods are inherently high in fat and devoid of carbohydrate and fiber. Given this diet, a sizable segment of the population will become overweight. They then make the mistake of reducing the *quantity* they eat, rather than abandoning the offensive foods. Many actually avoid carbohydrates because of the old myth that they are fattening. From the restrictive diets that result, cravings and binging can begin.

If children were raised on high-fiber, high-carbohydrate, vegetarian-based diets which are more modest in fat, weight problems would be much more rare, and diets would not be something most teenagers would consider.

The Size and Shape of Fat

Some of us come from families of heavy people and seem to gain weight by just thinking about food. Others have a natural tendency to be thin and cannot seem to gain weight no matter what. The mischievous hand of Mother Nature has played a role in overweight. Evidence suggests that a complex group of genetic factors can cause overweight to run in families.[10] These same studies show, however, that there is a large portion of the overweight problem that has nothing to do with genetics. We thought that our parents gave us a bad set of genes, when, in fact, they gave us a bad set of recipes and bad eating habits.

Shape is inherited as well. Some people are "pears." They tend to carry their weight in the hips and thighs. Others are "apples," tending to add weight in the abdomen. Some people are more cylindrical. The variety of shapes is nearly endless. "If you come from a family of apples, you're more likely to look like an apple," says Callaway. "Pear-shaped parents tend to have pear-shaped children. Even if you stay skinny, you can change your weight but you may not change your shape that much." In other words, you might become a skinny "pear," but you may still be a "pear." Some patterns of overweight are harder to reduce than others.

Also, some types of fat are more damaging to health than others. "Hip fat tends to come on with puberty and pregnancy," Callaway said. "It does not seem to come off as readily in response to either exercise or dieting as does belly fat. It doesn't look as if the hip and thigh fat is associated with diabetes, hypertension, high blood fats, or heart attacks."

This is different from abdominal fat, which comes on gradually in adulthood. Abdominal fat is easier to get rid of through food choices and physical activity. Getting rid of it is a good idea, because belly fat increases the risk of medical problems: diabetes, heart problems, high blood pressure, and even cancer of the uterus and ovary. In men, obesity leads to increased production of female sex hormones, which, in turn, can cause impotence; this can be reversed as weight is lost.

How much fat is medically dangerous? Measure around your waist and around your hips with a tape measure. For a man, increased risk of medical problems begins when his waist is larger than his hips. At that point, he definitely needs to lose weight. Women need a somewhat stricter criterion to avoid health problems; the waist should be no more than eighty percent of the hip measurement.

Overweight Children

Overweight children are not necessarily the victims of genetics. Weight problems can be the result of eating habits passed from one generation to the next. If they began a diet, they probably restricted the *quantity* of food, rather than making better food selections. They would slim down more effectively if their diets were modified to quite low-fat, essentially vegetarian diets, and if some regular physical activity were added.

"We frequently find that if we have an obese child, the parents are the same way," Connor said. "Unless they change, the kid won't change. Frequently they *don't* change. They may have soda pop, potato chips, ice cream, nuts, and cookies in the house all the time. The whole family needs to change its life-style."

Being an overweight kid is no fun. These children need help. Teasing and a sense of failure can pervade the developing self-image. If the family changes as a unit to healthier eating habits, the burden is taken off the children. There is a role played by genetics, but food choices and physical activity can be used intelligently to help make up for a tendency toward overweight.

Medical Conditions

Because overweight is so often wrongly regarded as a moral problem—a question of overindulgence and willpower— people seek dispensations on medical grounds. But if you had hoped to blame overweight on a medical condition, the fact is that they are rarely responsible. There are a few conditions in which medical problems lead to weight gain. In Cushing's syndrome, in which excess production of the hormone *cortisol* causes high blood pressure, fatigue, weakness, loss of menstrual periods, excess body hair, purplish abdominal discolorations, and other problems, overweight can occur, particularly in the torso. A few medications, such as steroids and anti-psychotic drugs, will cause an increase in appetite and require a bit of watching what one eats. But the vast majority of overweight people do not have a medical reason for their condition. "These conditions are extremely rare," Connor said. "Hypothyroidism used to be thought of as causing obesity. That isn't so. I haven't found anybody in my practice of about 35 years who was hypothyroid and overweight."

So, the bottom line is an optimistic one. Very few people have an unchangeable condition. Overweight people are victims, not of medical conditions for the most part, but of a set of food choices in combination with physical activity patterns and genetics. But now we know what to do. Instead of diets, we will tune up your metabolism, shift the menu to low-fat foods, and add physical activity to our daily lives.

What's Eating You?

Most overweight people do not continuously overindulge in vast quantities of foods. In fact, most eat less than thin people do. But some people do overeat on a regular basis. They keep eating well past the point when they are full. Some eat throughout the day. This can be for one of many reasons.

Some use food as an antidepressant or antianxiety drug. Food can be a pick-me-up for every stressor of the day. There is a special group of people, known as *carbohydrate cravers*, who eat large amounts of sugary or starchy snacks and are prone to depression, particularly in winter. As we'll see in Chapter 7, they may be using carbohydrates to boost a particular brain chemical, serotonin, which is known to play a role in combating depression.

For some people, food takes the place of something else that is missing. We require many forms of nourishment. In addition to food, we need social interactions, intellectual exercise, physical stimulation, sexual activity, rest and sleep, challenges in our lives, and some sense of success and mastery. For some of us, food becomes a substitute for one of these which is missing. Small children often have no more than a minimal interest in food, because their lives are filled with challenges and stimulation. If we can return these forms of "psychological nourishment" to our lives, we can be filled with more than just calories.

Some people who tend to overeat report that they do not feel in charge of themselves. They feel as if they are unable to control their weight. This control, they feel, is held by someone else: their doctor, a book, a magic formula. It is important to recognize these traits, because if you are one who feels out of control, then you would do well to make sure that your physician, family, and friends understand and support your efforts. You will be looking for their support and will respond to their encouragement. While you begin the long process of learning to trust yourself more, it helps to arrange social supports that can help you through your menu transition.

Some may use overweight as a defense. Fat distorts physique and blurs gender. Anxiety-provoking intimacies are far less likely when one has strayed a long way from one's normal weight. While the vast majority of overweight people are not in this category, for those who are, other means for handling the anxieties of interactions will have to be learned as the defense of fat is shed. Psychotherapy is useful in the process.

How does one know if there is a psychological contribution to obesity? Callaway says, "A clue to those folks is that they often are the 'stuffers.' They are among the 15 to 20 percent who are eating more than predicted and have higher than predicted metabolic rates. They often sweat a lot because they are generating a lot of heat. And when you ask, 'Why are you eating?' it's often for reasons other than hunger. There is no particular personality profile that you see in obesity, but there is a subgroup of people who are eating for other reasons, and it is important to identify that."

Steps To Weight Control

To permanently lose weight, you must permanently change the way you eat:

Increase carbohydrate. Grains, such as breads, rice, and pasta, legumes, such as beans and lentils, along with vegetables and fruits provide a satisfying, fiber-rich menu.

Get the fat off your plate. Meats, dairy products, poultry, fish, fried foods, and vegetable oils are the principal offenders. Trimming the fat from meat does not help very much; fat is marbled throughout meats. The key is to learn to prepare meat-free meals. The less fatty food you eat, the better.

Reduce consumption of concentrated sugars. While sugars are not as high in calories as fats are, they still contain more than we need and little else.

Include physical activity in your regular routine. Exercise burns calories and helps control your appetite. Choose something you enjoy so that it can become a permanent part of your life. Include a half-hour of physical activity each day.

Reset your metabolic rate. Carbohydrates help maintain an active metabolism. Exercise also raises your metabolic rate so you keep burning more calories even at rest, and it builds muscle, which in turn, also helps burn more calories. Avoid very-low-calorie diets. Include at least 10 calories in your daily menu for every pound you weigh currently. Distribute your calories in three meals a day.

Are you a starver, a skipper, or a stuffer? If you have been chronically dieting, you need to eat more calories, especially carbohydrates, to increase your metabolic rate. If you tend to skip meals, restore regular eating to avoid binging. If you are a stuffer, that is, a chronic overeater, a look at the reasons behind this behavior may be helpful.

Weight Control Checklist

Increase carbohydrate and fiber by choosing your menu from grains (breads, cereals, pasta, rice), beans, vegetables, and fruits (see also the recommendations in Chapter 10). These foods are modest in calories and boost your metabolism.

Decrease the fat content of your meals by eliminating meats, poultry, fish, added oils, and fried foods. Nuts and seeds should be kept to a minimum. Fatty foods are loaded with calories.

Avoid sugary foods and alcohol.

Include a half hour of exercise in your daily routine (under your doctor's supervision if you are over 40 or have any medical condition) to burn calories and boost your metabolism.

Enjoy three meals a day. Skipping meals slows down the metabolism.

Avoid diets which restrict caloric intake below ten calories per pound of current body weight. Diets slow the metabolism.

If you are "stuffing," that is, frequently overeating, you must take particular care to follow each of the above points very carefully. In addition, examine the circumstances in which overeating occurs.

The only factor in weight control you cannot change is your heredity. While this will affect both your size and your shape, you do have control over all of the above factors.

Chapter 5

Uninvited Guests: Food-Borne Illness

That "FLU" you had last winter may not have been the "flu" at all. It may have come from your supermarket's poultry department—one out of three chickens in the retail store carries live infectious salmonella bacteria. Or it might have come from a hamburger or a carton of eggs. Poultry, meat, and eggs at the supermarket have become "surprise packages," containing an unpredictable variety of contaminants: DDT and other pesticides, hormones, antibiotics, and live bacteria and other organisms that may cause millions of cases of "flu"-like illness every year in the U.S.

Salmonella

In January, 1983, a young man in Minnesota became very ill. He had an intestinal illness that was so serious that hospitalization was necessary. But his doctors found that what he had was actually not a typical viral "flu." It was an infection with salmonella, a type of bacteria often found in poultry and other meat products. Where he picked up salmonella was not clear at first. All that was certain was that he had fever and diarrhea and was very sick.

The young man was the first case in the Minnesota outbreak. Another case of salmonella infection turned up in a

33-year-old woman. More and more people became ill. The youngest patient was eight; the oldest, 43. In many cases, before the illness began, the patients had been using antibiotics for an unrelated illness, such as bronchitis or an ear infection. Health officials first thought a contaminated antibiotic must have been spreading the disease. But the patients had all been using different antibiotic preparations. The bacteria were not in the pills. But where were they coming from?

A team from the Centers for Disease Control investigated.[1,2] They found that many of the patients had eaten hamburger which had come from a particular farm in South Dakota. Beef from the farm had been sent to a vocational school which trained butchers and to meat brokers who distributed products to several supermarkets. The beef carried live salmonella. Next to the beef farm was a dairy farm, where the salmonella "bug" killed a calf and then infected a young farmer.

One unfortunate man was drawn into the outbreak without eating any tainted beef at all. He was in the hospital for an abdominal injury and was examined with a sigmoidoscope which had last been used on one of the patients with salmonella. The scope had been treated with a disinfectant, but it transmitted the bacteria to the man, who then died from a massive salmonella infection.

Another outbreak, this time in California, was reported in the *New England Journal of Medicine* in March, 1987.[3] The source was a herd of dairy cows who had routinely been fed antibiotics as a growth-promoter. The cows had become infected with salmonella. The infection was very difficult to treat because the bacteria had developed a resistance to the antibiotics the farmer had been using all along. So rather than fight an uphill battle against the bacteria, the farmer simply sold the cattle to slaughter. The meat ended up in fast-food restaurants and supermarkets, where it caused a serious outbreak.

Nowadays, salmonella contamination is an everyday event. Millions of people every year have what they believe is a viral illness, but which actually came in the door with their groceries. The bacteria are often found in chicken, turkey, beef, pork, and other animal products. Why? For three reasons: the first is the way farm animals are raised. The second is the fact that the meat inspection system cannot detect salmonella. Finally, under federal regulations, it is perfectly legal to sell salmonella-tainted products.

We like to think of our food products as coming to us in pristine packages produced under immaculate conditions, carefully monitored by trained government inspectors. Unfortunately, this is hardly the case. Take poultry, for example: modern farm operations raise chickens as if they were popcorn. A few thousand tiny chicks are put into a large steel building, and the doors are closed. Eight weeks later, thousands of big, round, fluffy, white birds are shoulder-to-shoulder, ready to be sold to slaughter. Unlike popcorn, however, they have been producing excrement continuously. In the cramped factory-farm design, there is nowhere they can go to get out of it.

As Assistant Secretary of Agriculture, Carol Tucker Foreman was responsible for the meat inspection system during the Carter Administration. She was gravely concerned that consumers were being routinely sold meat products that contained contaminants of all sorts and that the government had done little to stop it.

"Chickens are dirty animals," Foreman said. "Turkeys are dirty animals. When they are raised in close confinement, any filth that they pick up is going to be transferred from one bird to another. There are thousands of birds in a chicken house. You can imagine, they just live on a bed of feces. Their droppings are all over the place. They peck at their own droppings. They peck at each other. To the extent they fall down they get covered with feces."

One might hope that chicken houses would be cleaned occasionally, but the cramped conditions of the modern chicken operation are more like a factory than a farm. No one could possibly sweep around the birds during the growing season.

"'Would you stand on your left leg please?'" Forman laughed. "If you pass by a chicken house in the summertime, you feel fairly confident that they don't clean them out very often. They clean the floor at the end of the raising of each flock, if then."

Most operations, in fact, clean their buildings only about once a year, so for their whole lives the chickens are walking through their accumulating excrement.

"They're then brought to the slaughterhouse." Foreman said. "Chickens are hung upside down and slaughtered, and then their feathers are beaten and hosed off. The beating process that dislodges the feathers tends to beat into the skin of the chicken any feces or other dirt that they happen to have on them. So instead of getting it off, it's beaten in."

A former executive director of the Consumer Federation of America, Carol Tucker Foreman came from Arkansas with a good-natured directness and an uncompromising demand for safety. Her description of the disease-ridden meat industry is reminiscent of Upton Sinclair's classic condemnation of the Chicago slaughterhouses, *The Jungle*. Chickens not already covered with salmonella are likely to be contaminated as they go through the slaughterhouse.

"You have a production line that's run at a very rapid speed," Foreman said. "The chickens are eviscerated. If you've got real fancy equipment, you can run the line very, very fast and never puncture an intestine. But if your equipment is a little old or isn't adjusted just right, you'll puncture the intestines on large numbers of birds, and then the feces contaminate the birds.

"The last big place in the line where they get that contamination is when they put the poultry through a water bath. After all, it's a dead bird. It's a warm animal. In order to keep it from spoiling, you have to reduce its temperature very rapidly. They put it into a bath of very cold water. Any filth that's on the bird gets put into the bath water.

"Under the USDA rules, if there are feces on a bird, you can use all the meat if you wash the bird with chlorinated water. These days I would probably require both cutting [off the contaminated part] and washing because the salmonella level is too high. It's not enough to say that a particular process doesn't increase the contamination level. You ought to be looking for a process that decreases it.

"The Germans and the Common Market countries have now begun requiring a spin-drum process. American producers don't want to do that for a variety of reasons, not the least of which is that chickens are very absorbent animals. When you put them into the water bath to chill them they gain a little weight. Since chicken is sold by the pound, over a period of time it's a substantial financial difference to the company. The average broiler is about four pounds. If you can add a quarter of a pound or an eighth of a pound in water pickup, that's very important to the economics of the industry."

The water and juice in chicken packages has been called "fecal soup." It is often loaded with disease-causing salmonella and other bacteria. Why doesn't inspection pick up the bacterial contamination? Because salmonella bacteria are not visible to the naked eye.

"You can't see salmonella," Foreman said. "Inspection is done in a horse-and-buggy way. There are four billion chickens slaughtered each year, and each one of them is examined by a warm human being. They take a bird and they kind of feel a leg and a wing at the same time, and they look at the back, and they turn it and look at the front, and then they tilt it and look into the body cavity and feel the viscera. Inspectors look for obvious filth, for abscesses and tumors, and for broken bones, which I've never been sure is terribly important to consumers. They place a high premium on having a plant that's clean and a bird that looks good at the end of the line. Only one or two diseases

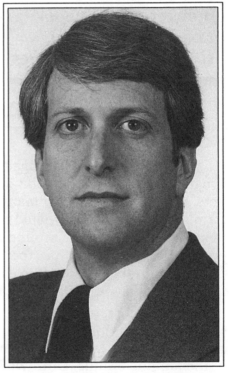

Dr. Mitchell Cohen

that make chickens sick cause humans to be ill. But because poultry inspection was initially intended for the improvement of the animal stock, those were the things that inspectors concentrated on. You can't see salmonella. You can see things like feces that you assume are associated with it, but you can't see the salmonella. It may be much more extensive than any filth you can see.

"In addition, you can't see antibiotics or other chemical residues. If the animal has somehow come in touch with PCBs or DDT or Aldrin or Dieldrin or any of about 70 or so other chemicals that USDA tests for on a random sampling basis, the inspector has no way of seeing that, and there is no way that they will be able to see it in the near future. There's no way to make sure that a given bird isn't contaminated with salmonella or DDT. We just keep spending money doing the things that we know how to do, but that may not be important anymore."

> *"People have gone to the store and picked up packages of poultry and taken them off to a laboratory and checked them for salmonella contamination. The number of birds contaminated has been shown in several studies to be around a third."*
>
> *Carol Tucker Foreman*

As the chicken is packaged and sent to the supermarket, it carries the live salmonella along. Studies have looked at how often chicken is contaminated with salmonella. "The number of birds contaminated by salmonella has been shown in several studies to be around a third," Foreman said. "The people have gone to the store and picked up packages of poultry and taken them off to a laboratory and checked them for salmonella contamination. About a third."

Can the customer know that a certain brand of chicken is safe? Foreman remarked, "No, because if you went to the store and checked you would find salmonella contamination in any of the famous brands. Until we know more about preventing salmonella contamination and until the way USDA does inspection is changed, the public will have to be very, very careful about how they handle chicken.

"One of the big reasons that the incidence of salmonella poisoning in the United States is increasing these days is that we eat a lot more chicken than we used to," Foreman said. "We eat a lot of it in delicatessen settings. Making chicken salad in a mass operation is an invitation to salmonella. You put mayonnaise and chicken together with a little salmonella in it, and if the temperature gets a bit too high, you're going to have an enormous multiplication of the bacteria."

Salmonella illness often masquerades as the "flu," with vomiting, diarrhea, crampy abdominal pain and low-grade fever. It begins within 6 to 48 hours after ingestion of contaminated food. Usually, the illness passes within several days without treatment, but sometimes it persists and becomes very serious. It may spread through the blood to infect the bones, joints, lungs, liver, kidney, or the membranes that surround the heart and brain. And in thousands of cases each year, it is fatal.

> *"One of the big reasons that the incidence of salmonella poisoning in the United States is increasing these days is that we eat a lot more chicken than we used to."*
>
> **Carol Tucker Foreman**

"It is a significant problem," said Mitchell Cohen, M.D., of the Centers for Disease Control in Atlanta. The CDC is the focal point where information on contagious illnesses is gathered and from which investigations into outbreaks are directed. They have found that the reported cases of salmonella are only the tip of the iceberg.

"It's been estimated that salmonellosis costs patients and producers over a billion dollars each year," Cohen said, "and that the reported cases only represent one-tenth to one-hundredth of the actual number of cases. There are probably between 400,000 and four million cases of salmonellosis a year in the United States."

Who should be concerned? The high fever, diarrhea, meningitis, infections of bones, joints, and the blood that can occur from salmonella illness are not treats for anyone. It can be quite serious, especially among the elderly. But there is another group at even more risk, the highest incidence being in three-month-old babies. All too often, diarrhea and fever in infants is caused by salmonella.

Of course, small babies do not eat chicken. How do they get salmonella? Raw meat can pass infectious bacteria onto any surface it touches. A mother may wipe up chicken juice from the counter top and later wipe off her baby's pacifier with the same sponge. The pacifier goes in the baby's mouth along with the infectious salmonella bacteria. Or simply touching raw chicken or other meat can pass bacteria which can survive on the hands for several hours. Salmonella can also infect an adult and then

> *"We have had outbreaks of salmonella related to almost every food of animal origin: poultry, beef, pork, eggs, milk, and milk products."*
>
> **Dr. Mitchell Cohen**

be passed to a child. "Cross-contamination is the most serious problem with salmonella," Foreman said. "If you open a package of chicken on the counter and pick the pieces out, there's always some water and meat juice in the bottom of the container. You cut the chicken up on a cutting board, a wooden cutting board for example, and then wipe the counter clean with a sponge and toss the sponge into the sink. Salmonella just love a sponge. And then they get passed on to the tabletop or to utensils or to anything else that you might use the sponge on. Or you may use that cutting board to cut up vegetables."

Cohen adds, "It's likely that the organisms are brought into the household, for example, through contaminated chicken, and are transferred to food preparation surfaces or utensils and eventually to the infant's formula. There also can be direct transmission to an infant from a person who has been infected. Salmonellosis in the very young or old can be a very serious illness."

All this from bringing chicken into the household? Salmonella is not only found in chickens. Any animal product can be contaminated, as Dr. Cohen points out. "We have had outbreaks of salmonella related to almost every food of animal origin: poultry, beef, pork, eggs, milk, and milk products."

Salmonella can even get inside an egg. Again, the problem is the intensely crowded conditions of the modern factory-farm, where chickens literally live in each others feces. In the 1960s, egg products used in baking frequently caused outbreaks of disease. It also became clear that salmonella on the surface of an egg could get inside if the shell were cracked. But there have been increasing reports of intact grade A eggs harboring live salmonella, causing thousands of cases of illness.[4] The bacteria pass into the eggs while still inside the chicken, and evidently can also pass through the shell from external contamination.

Foreman dealt with outbreaks in her work at the Department of Agriculture. "The worst salmonella contamination that we dealt with while I was at USDA," she said, "was from rare roast beef sandwiches that were sold at delis all over the country, but especially in New York, New Jersey, and Philadelphia. These little lunch rooms in the basements of office buildings don't cook things like roast beef on premises. They buy roast beef from a central kitchen. To keep it rare, the temperature never goes high enough for a long enough period of time to kill the salmonella. It's then wrapped, sent out on a truck and delivered. It may sit on a cooler counter that's not quite cool enough, and then somebody may buy the sandwich and wait a couple of hours before they eat it. Those incidents in the late seventies were reported frequently."

The Department of Agriculture stepped in and addressed the problem. "I, however," said Foreman, "never eat rare roast beef sandwiches from somebody's delicatessen."

"People have to appreciate that there are certain high-risk food items," Cohen said. "Foods of animal origin are likely to be contaminated with salmonella."

All animal products are potential sources of salmonella. Steps that can help prevent salmonella infection are detailed at the end of this chapter.

The Antibiotic Connection

Cattle, chickens, and other animals often carry salmonella and other bacteria in their intestinal tracts. Farmers now routinely aggravate this problem by feeding low doses of antibiotics to their animals. The farmer is not using the antibiotics to kill off invading bacteria. The doses farmers use are *subtherapeutic*, that is, insufficient to counter infections. The antibiotics are used to make the animals grow faster, increasing the farmer's profit margin. For reasons no one fully understands, antibiotics promote the growth of the animals. In the process, they foster the growth of bacteria that can resist antibiotics. New strains of bacteria develop in these animals, strains that are very hard to control. When they infect animals or people, our usual antibiotics may be entirely ineffective.

Antibiotics in livestock feeds have given bacteria the upper hand in human illness. If antibiotic-resistant salmonella are eaten in food, they can remain dormant in the intestinal tract, held in check by the normal intestinal bacteria. But if antibiotics are then used for some other condition, they will kill off the normal gut bacteria that had held the salmonella in check. The salmonella can resist the antibiotics, and then overgrow and cause a very serious illness.

"A quarter or more of salmonella are now resistant to commonly used antibiotics," Cohen said. "In a recent report, a person died because she was treated with what was thought to be the drug of choice. The organism was subsequently found to be resistant to that antibiotic."

> "A quarter or more of salmonella are now resistant to commonly used antibiotics."
>
> **Dr. Mitchell Cohen**

Because the indiscriminate use of antibiotics promotes the growth of resistant bacteria, doctors now avoid using antibiotics unless clearly necessary. But antibiotics are a routine ingredient in animal agriculture.

"If you go to your pediatrician or your internist with a little sore throat," Foreman said, "they don't give you penicillin until they're sure it's a bacterial and not a viral infection. They don't want to overuse penicillin. And yet two-thirds or three-quarters of all of the penicillin and tetracycline manufactured in this country go for subtherapeutic use in animal production. As a matter of course, poultry, cattle, and hogs in this country are raised on feed that is medicated. American Cyanamid doesn't make its profits selling antibiotics for human beings; they make it selling antibiotics for animals."

In 1977, the Food and Drug Administration proposed eliminating the subtherapeutic use of penicillin and tetracycline in animal feed. But just as the sympathies for farmers have led Congress to subsidize tobacco crops and dairy products, Congress also has not allowed restrictions on antibiotics used to promote animal growth.

Other Organisms in Foods

Campylobacter is another unpleasant surprise often found in poultry. The National Research Council called it "one of the most common bacterial causes of gastroenteritis among both children and adults."[5] Like salmonella, it simulates a viral "flu," with nausea and vomiting, diarrhea, abdominal pain, and fever. Occasionally, it is mistaken for appendicitis. Small children are the most frequent victims of campylobacter.

Campylobacter is carried into the slaughterhouse with chickens or other animals and is spread around further in the process of slaughter, "cleaning," and cooling. Some estimates have put the contamination rate as high as 65 to 80 percent.[6,7] Many strains are resistant to commonly used antibiotics. As a result, at least two million cases of campylobacter infection occur every year in the U.S. USDA inspector Hobart Bartley said, "If the American public knew what garbage they were eating, they would revolt."

"Two-thirds or three quarters of all of the penicillin and tetracycline manufactured in this country go for subtherapeutic use in animal production. As a matter of course, poultry, cattle, and hogs in this country are raised on feed that is medicated."

Carol Tucker Foreman

Yersinia enterocolitica is an unfriendly "bug" lurking in pork, contaminated milk, and, in rare cases, spring water. Like campylobacter, illness from yersinia can masquerade as appendicitis, and causes diarrhea, fever, abdominal pain, and vomiting, particularly in children.[8]

Another common contaminant is listeria (*listeria monocytogenes*). It has been the cause of hundreds of product recalls, particularly of dairy products. Processed meats and shellfish have also been sources of contamination. Although healthy people are usually resistant to infection, the elderly or chronically ill are often at risk of an intestinal illness which can spread to the blood stream and brain. Fetuses are often killed by the bacteria.

Birth defects can come from foods. *Toxoplasma* is a protozoan (one-celled animal) present in 30 percent of pork products, ten percent of lamb, and in many other animal products. The most common source of toxoplasma is undercooked or raw meat. In addition, cross-contamination of food-handling surfaces can occur. Millions of people are infected with toxoplasma with no problem at all. But if a woman acquires toxoplasmosis during pregnancy, her baby is at risk for birth defects, including blindness and brain damage.

What these contaminants have in common is a tendency to be present in foods of animal origin and to attack most viciously those who are very young or old or who are compromised by other illnesses.

Poison-Producing Bacteria

Everyone has heard of botulism. *Clostridium botulinum* bacteria, typically in canned foods, produce a potent toxin that causes blurred vision, weakness, and possibly even death. Happily, commercial canners are very careful to prevent such contamination, and there are now only about 30 cases of botulism per year in the U.S., mainly due to home canning.

There are other poison-producing bacteria that find their way into foods. *Staphylococci* (or "staph"), for example, normally live on human skin. Another, called *Clostridium perfringens*, normally lives in the human intestinal tract. Generally, these bacteria do no harm. They are a part of our environment. But when allowed to incubate in warm foods, they can cause problems. Both of these bacteria flourish in high-protein foods. When they are allowed to sit in foods for several hours at room temperature, staph produce a chemical poison. Nausea, vomiting, and diarrhea result within two to four hours of eating the contaminated food.

"What typically happens," Cohen said, "is that a person who is harboring this organism contaminates the food, and the food is left out so that the bacteria replicate and produce the toxin. Then other people consume it. This is a frequent problem at picnics or banquets where there may be a good opportunity for foods to sit out." In the case of the staph toxin, cooking the food again will not help. The toxin is not destroyed by heat.

Similarly, clostridia spores may get into foods through poor hygiene. These spores are not killed by cooking. Instead, cooking actually heat-shocks them, causing them to become active bacteria which produce a toxin. If the food is then eaten, a "flu"-like illness is the result. This toxin is, however, sensitive to heat. If the food is cooked again, the toxin will be destroyed along with the bacteria.

E. coli

In January, 1993, food poisoning reached a new and grotesque level. That was the beginning of the Jack-in-the-Box disaster. A new bacterium, called E. coli 0157:H7, had caused its first disease outbreak 11 years earlier, soon followed by several others. E. coli is found in cow feces. During slaughter and processing, it contaminates meat and is undetected by government meat inspectors, who check only the appearance of meat and do not routinely use bacterial tests. On January 10, 1993, a two-year-old-boy in Tacoma, Washington, ate a cheeseburger at a Jack-in-the-Box restaurant. The next day he developed fever and vomiting. On January 13, he was hospitalized. Nine days later, he was dead.

The Jack-in-the-Box restaurant chain in several western states sold ground beef that looked and tasted normal, but made 600 children and adults seriously ill. Hospitalization was necessary for 144 of them. Three children and one adult died.

The U.S. Department of Agriculture rushed in. Secretary Mike Espy and others held hearings, promising aggressive new programs. But it soon became clear the Department of

Agriculture's main interest was not in cleaning up meat products, but rather in cleaning up the image of American agriculture, while brushing aside consumer worries. A year later, virtually nothing had been done to correct the problem. And on January 8, 1994, a thirteen-year-old boy in Aberdeen, Washington, had a burger at a fast food restaurant. Fifteen days later he was dead. His parents thought the E. coli problem must have been solved, because the government had seemingly given it so much attention. But they learned a bitter lesson. The government is doing virtually nothing to stop it Federal officials estimate there may be as many as 20,000 cases of E. coli infection every year.

E. coli 0517:H7 infections come mainly from beef and raw milk, and from water contaminated by animal wastes. Like salmonella, it is easily transmitted by kitchen surfaces and utensils, and by person-to-person contact. Illness is caused, not by the bacterium itself, but by a toxin it produces. Symptoms range from mild diarrhea to severe cramps with bloody diarrhea. Some cases progress to the hemolytic uremic syndrome (HUS) in which the bacterial toxin destroys blood cells and platelets, and damages the kidneys and other organs. About five to ten percent of those with HUS die. Current antibiotics and antimotility drugs are useless against E. coli 0157:H7 and may even worsen the disease.

A Department of Agriculture survey tested beef carcasses between October, 1992, and November, 1993. Disease-causing bacteria, including clostridia, campylobacter, staphylococci, listeria, salmonella, and, yes, E. coli 0157:H7, were found on 15 percent of them.[9] There is no reason to expect this problem to get better any time soon, and it is yet another reason to steer clear of animal products.

Raw Bar Roulette

Oysters are eaten straight from the shell at raw bars. Raw fish are often a part of Japanese cuisine. Hygiene, however, is not their strong suit.

In April, 1988, the Food and Drug Administration sent out a warning to physicians about the dangers of raw shellfish.[10] Contamination by the bacteria *Vibrio vulnificus* was widespread, especially in oysters. People with liver disease, alcoholism, cancer, blood diseases, AIDS, and AIDS-related complex are at particular risk for the damage these bacteria can do. The FDA estimated that the bacteria were present in 5 to 10 percent of raw shellfish on the market. And there are no known methods for separating infected shellfish from those free of infection.

"If you decide that you want to eat raw shellfish," Cohen said, "you're exposing yourself to whatever disease-causing bacteria that that shellfish may have been exposed to, from human sewage, as well as to bacteria which occur naturally in the shellfish's environment. People can get hepatitis, salmonellosis, or cholera from consuming shellfish that have been contaminated with human waste. In addition, some disease-causing bacteria are normally present in unpolluted environments."

In his work at the CDC, Dr. Cohen has no appetite for raw oysters. "When I look at certain foods," he said, "I think about how the foods are handled and whether or not something is likely to be potentially hazardous. To me, consuming raw shellfish isn't worth the risk. There are no benefits to outweigh the risks."

Concerns extend to other kinds of raw fish. Cohen adds, "In assuming that raw fish is safe you are making several additional assumptions: that the person who prepared it has handled it appropriately, that they know how to recognize parasites, that after it's been prepared it's not been in conditions that would favor bacterial growth. In Japan the most common cause of food poisoning is *Vibrio parahemolyticus*, which is a bacterial infection that is transmitted through raw fish and shellfish. So even in an area where the people are very skillful in dealing with these foods, there is still significant occurrence of disease."

Infectious bacteria and parasites are not the only problems in fish. Chemicals are often disposed of by being discarded in waterways. As a result, fish often become contaminated. In addition, as small fish are consumed by larger fish, contaminants tend to become more and more concentrated. Yet the fish industry is the most poorly inspected of all the meat industries. There is essentially no way of assuring the safety of available fish products.

DDT and Other
Three-Letter Words

All sorts of chemicals find their way into foods. Our inspectors do not have ways of checking for them all. But even for those that can be detected, however, the foods are rarely removed from the market. The monitoring process does not generally report on samples until after the remaining foods have been sold and consumed.[5] "You may find out two weeks later that it was just laden with DDT," Foreman said. "By that time the meat's been eaten."

DDT is not used in this country any more. It was banned in 1972, although sporadic use of the chemical continued in the next few years. But DDT remains in the environment. Since its widespread use as a sprayed pesticide, it circulates widely in the atmosphere. As it settles on the soil it becomes part of plants and, particularly, of animals who concentrate the chemical in their fatty tissues. Is DDT still found in meat?

"Sure," Foreman said. "It's one of the residues that they find most frequently. DDT is ubiquitous. Once it's in the atmosphere, it stays there for a very long time. If there's ground that's contaminated with DDT, the corn grown or stored near that ground comes out contaminated with DDT and the animals may be contaminated with it.

"Nobody knows how much DDT you have to have to be sick from it or what the impact may be a generation from now or two generations from now. I think that warrants a very conservative approach. If you don't know what the impact is likely to be or if you don't know from how many sources you may get a particular contaminant, then you ought to do everything possible to make sure that you're as free from the contamination as you possibly can be. We've been almost in the reverse situation for a long time, requiring clear proof that chemicals are harmful before doing anything."

In addition, chemicals banned for use in this country can, in some cases, continue to be manufactured for export. Agricultural products which are then imported into the U.S. may carry these chemicals back into our food supply.

PCBs

Polychlorinated biphenyls (PCBs) were manufactured for use in electrical transformers and other commercial applications. From this humble beginning, PCBs have achieved notoriety as some of the most poisonous chemicals ever produced.

"We had thousands of chickens and eggs contaminated with PCBs which had leaked out of an unused transformer into a pit where meat by-products were being kept," Foreman said. "They were then turned into chicken feed, and the chickens that ate the feed were all contaminated with PCBs. As late as 1979 or 1980, electrical transformers with PCBs in them were still being used in food plants all over the country."

PCBs cause cancer. Acute exposure can cause liver damage and a variety of other symptoms. PCBs are easily passed from a nursing mother to her breast-fed infant.

Although manufacture of the chemicals was banned in 1979, getting rid of them continues to be a major problem. PCBs have often been found in fish, as a result of leakage or intentional dumping of PCBs into waterways. A 1987 study, conducted by Laval University in Quebec, showed that Eskimo women have PCB concentrations in their breast milk that are more than double the tolerance levels set by the Canadian government. These concentrations are sufficient to cause serious illnesses in their nursing infants. The cause is the fish-based Eskimo diet. PCBs can spread many, many miles from the dumping site. Researchers at Wayne State University in Detroit found that women eating Lake Michigan fish only two or three times per month gave birth to children who were sluggish, had smaller head circumferences and lower birth weights compared to the children of mothers who ate less (or no) fish. "I would advise women of child-bearing age not to eat fatty fish like salmon and lake trout at all," said Joseph L. Jacobsen, one of the Wayne State researchers. The problem was PCBs passed from the fish to the women who ate them. PCBs can remain in the body for prolonged periods of time, a stock-pile of toxins waiting to damage a developing baby. Birds, such as ducks and geese, that feed on these fish may also be highly contaminated. In addition, PCB contamination of animal feeds has spread the chemical to meats and eggs.

Hormones and Other Chemicals

Diethylstilbestrol (DES) is a synthetic female sex hormone which was used to prevent miscarriage. Women exposed to DES when they were babies have now grown up to find themselves at increased risk for cervical and vaginal cancer. DES is no longer used for that purpose, but DES and related chemicals have occasionally reached the consumer through meat products. They have been used to fatten up livestock. A small implant in a steer's ear is gradually absorbed and promotes growth. The amounts of DES received by consumers in meats were large enough to raise concerns about their cancer-causing potential and their ability to alter the sexual maturation of children.

"The FDA finally succeeded in late 1979 in getting the manufacture or sale of DES for use in animal products banned," Foreman said. "There's some evidence that there is a black market—not of very large proportion—but some evidence of a black market in DES. We had a case in 1980 where a farmer raised a complaint because he was mad at his business partners. He said, 'Those guys are all out there using DES.' FDA went out to investigate and sure enough there were all these herds that had implants of DES."

The use of other growth-promoting hormones is still legal. But these chemicals are only a small fraction of the problem. There are many, many other contaminants. "Insecticides, pesticides, products that are used in paint and preservation of wood that may have harmful chemicals in them, hormones, and animal drugs all turn up in meat," Foreman said. "Sulfa is the worst drug in terms of residue violations. It's used heavily

> *"Insecticides, pesticides, products that are used in paint and preservation of wood, hormones, and animal drugs all turn up in meat."*
>
> **Carol Tucker Foreman**

in pork production in medicated feed. It causes some people to break out in a rash.

Chemicals on Fruits and Vegetables

Produce is routinely sprayed with pesticides and other agricultural chemicals.[11,12] Unfortunately, many of these chemicals are carcinogenic, toxic to nerves, or poisonous in other ways. Children consume far more fruits than do adults, and they are more vulnerable to the toxic effects of chemicals. Tomatoes, potatoes, apples, citrus fruits, and many other fruits and vegetables are frequently treated with chemicals which they carry along to the produce department.

Fortunately, there are ways to minimize our risk. Unlike the chemical contaminants in meats or milk which are permeated throughout the product, the chemicals on produce are usually on the surface. Peeling fruits and vegetables is often helpful. All produce should be washed. A dilute soap solution and plenty of water will help remove some chemical residues. Waxes cannot be washed off, and waxed produce should be peeled.

When buying produce, ask for organically grown produce. Most health food stores carry a good selection. Avoid non-domestic produce, since it may have been treated with chemicals now banned in the U.S. Of course, some people grow vegetables of their own.

Are inadvertent exposures to chemicals through foods responsible for birth defects or for childhood leukemias? Recent studies have shown that chemicals used around the home and the workplace can put children at risk. Whether the insecticides or other chemicals that turn up in foods are also responsible for birth defects or childhood cancers is not known.

"Since the mid-1940s, we've used chemicals extensively in agricultural production," Foreman said. "We used them in willy-nilly fashion without testing them first. They were viewed as a great benefit to mankind, and no one asked what are the unintended consequences."

Thanks, But No Thanks

As problematic as chemical residues on produce may be, chemicals in meats are even more difficult to deal with. These chemicals cannot be washed or peeled from meats as they sometimes can from produce.

Meats must be regarded as carrying live infectious bacteria, parasites, and chemical residues. Although both Foreman and Cohen believe that correct handling and cooking can minimize the chances that bacteria or parasites will survive in the kitchen, bringing these products into the home always poses a risk of contamination.

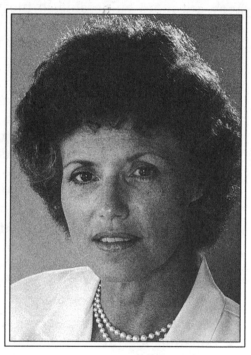

Carol Tucker Foreman

The surest way to avoid chemical contamination is to decline the dubious honor of being at the top of the food chain. If plants contain a low-level of chemical contamination, animals who eat them will concentrate these chemicals. If these animals are, in turn, eaten by others (or by humans), a progressive increase in the level of contamination occurs. By choosing plant foods, we find less contamination.

At the very top of the food chain is the human infant. The breast-fed infant is the target, not only of the contamination ingested by his or her mother, but of her tendency to further concentrate chemicals in her fatty tissues, such as breast tissue. According to a study at Colorado State University, published in the *New England Journal of Medicine*, vegetarian mothers have far lower levels of chemical contaminants in their breast milk than non-vegetarians.[13] The more our diet relies on foods from plants, rather than from animals, the less contamination we will encounter. The more we know about the foods we eat, the better able we will be to protect ourselves.

Steps For Safe Cooking

How can we avoid contracting bacterial illnesses such as salmonella and campylobacter? How can we keep chemical exposures off our dinner plates?

1. *Suspect all raw animal products.* Animal products must be regarded as carrying live bacteria. There is no nutritional reason to consume meats, eggs, or any other animal product. Those who avoid them have considerably less risk of food contamination.

2. *Cook food adequately.* For those who consume animal products, all meats must be thoroughly cooked. Meats that are raw or poorly cooked can harbor live bacteria. Eggs must be boiled for seven minutes, poached for five minutes, or fried for three minutes on each side. Cooking eggs "sunny-side up" cannot kill salmonella, no matter how long the cooking continues.[14] Avoid products that use raw eggs or nearly raw eggs: Caesar salad dressing, hollandaise sauce, eggnog, homemade ice cream. Phase animal products out of your diet is the best approach.

3. *Avoid contaminating food after it is cooked.* Bacteria can easily get into food after it is cooked. Only very hot or very cold temperatures prevent multiplication of bacteria: less than 40 degrees or greater than 140 degrees Fahrenheit.

4. *Prevent cross-contamination.* Wash hands and any surface raw animal products have touched, including counter tops, sponges, and utensils. Avoid using wooden cutting boards for any meat items.

5. *Chemical contaminants cannot be removed from meats.*

6. *Buy organically grown fruits and vegetables whenever possible.* Chemically treated produce should be washed for two minutes in a dilute detergent solution, then thoroughly rinsed. Peels should be removed.

Chapter 6

Other Common Health Problems

Are varicose veins, appendicitis, or gallstones related to what we eat? Believe it or not, the answer is yes. Surprising links are being found between dietary factors and many common health problems. Constipation, hemorrhoids, hiatus hernia, diabetes, osteoporosis, kidney disease, and even impotence are among the other common problems related to foods. In this chapter, we will take a brief look at these connections. The story begins, not in the United States, but in Africa.

Denis Burkitt and Fiber

For 20 years, Denis Burkitt, M.D., practiced surgery in Africa. An adventurous and widely traveled man, Burkitt achieved fame in medicine for identifying and curing a form of childhood cancer now known as Burkitt's lymphoma, the first human cancer shown to be caused by a virus (see Chapter 3).

On the heels of this important work, Burkitt began to notice that many common Western diseases were conspicuous by their absence in Africa. For example, while there might be two cases of appendicitis a day in the major hospitals of Western countries, Burkitt found only about two cases *per year* among Africans. Many other illnesses were also extraordinarily rare wherever modern food preparation methods had not been put to use.

"I was doing ward rounds in English hospitals and American hospitals," Burkitt said, "and it struck me that all the beds were full of patients suffering from diseases I didn't see in Africa: coronary heart disease, the commonest cause of death; gallstones, the commonest abdominal operation; appendicitis, the commonest abdominal emergency; varicose veins and hemorrhoids, the commonest venous disorders; colorectal cancer, the second commonest cancer death; diverticular disease, one of the commonest disorders of the gut; hiatus hernia, one of the commonest disorders of the stomach. It seems as if we have in front of us the mass of disease, which has to be preventable. I said to myself, if it really is possible to prevent our common diseases, why are we spending our time treating them?"

He took an interest in the hypothesis of a retired naval physician named Captain Cleave that many diseases common to Western countries were the result of overly refined foods, especially sugar and white flour. While Cleave had only found a piece of the puzzle, it was enough to get Burkitt going.

Burkitt came to find that refined sugar was by no means the whole explanation. A critical factor is fiber. In the modern refining methods used for grains, the fiber—the portion of vegetable foods that resists digestion—is discarded. In the process, the fiber content of the diet drops dramatically. At the same time, vegetables, beans, and fruits have become second-class foods, while meat and dairy products have become a larger and larger part of our routine. As the high-fat, low-fiber diet takes hold around the world, Africa, India, and Asian countries that have never known Western diseases see an increasing occurrence of epidemics of diabetes, obesity, appendicitis, colon cancer, and heart disease following successively like a funeral procession.

Burkitt was not the first person to be interested in fiber. Hippocrates used whole grains as medical treatments. The Kellogg brothers in America had been proponents of the health benefits of cereal grains.

"And there was an interesting chap in the 1920s called Arbuthnot Lane," Burkitt said. "He was a surgeon. And he got the concept that most ills were due to stagnation of the fecal content in the colon. So being a surgeon, he thought the best thing to do was to cut out the colon. He thought it would be a good thing if all children had their colons cut out early in life, and then they would be exempt from all sorts of problems! He cut out the colon for all kinds of conditions. And then he suddenly came to the conclusion that it was much easier to give bran than to cut out the colon, and it had the same effect. So he gave up cutting out the colon and gave people bran instead."

As cultures undergo a Westernization of diet—for example, Japanese or Africans coming to America, or Asians adopting a Western diet within their own countries—diseases emerge in a certain order. Some are seen very soon; others only after many years. Interestingly, these diseases appear in the changing population in about the same order as they develop in individuals. For example, obesity becomes evident well before heart attacks.

"Diabetes is unknown in undomesticated animals," Burkitt said. "It's the commonest endocrine disease in Western man, and it's one of the first diseases that comes in after a change in life-style. Obesity comes in early. Appendicitis not quite so early, probably a decade or two later. But we've never seen gallstones or coronary heart disease emerge until about thirty years after diabetes becomes common. You never find coronary heart disease in a culture without diabetes.

> *"Diabetes is the commonest endocrine disease in Western man, and it's one of the first diseases that comes in after a change in lifestyle."*
>
> **Denis Burkitt**

"After the second World War, the government helped to feed the Pima Indians of Arizona," Burkitt said. "They suddenly plunged into popcorn, french fries, and hamburgers. They have the highest rate of gallstones in the world now and the second highest rate of diabetes, after the people on the island of Nauru who suddenly became millionaires overnight and changed their whole life-style." The traditional diet of the these Indians—desert legumes, with occasional cacti, fish, and seeds—has been shown to be superior from a health perspective than the foods the government has unloaded on them.[1] Meanwhile, in parts of rural Africa where a Westernized diet has not yet taken hold, these chronic diseases are still rare. Childhood illnesses, particularly infections, do occur, but the Western diet-related diseases are very uncommon. As a result, many adult Africans live to a ripe old age.

"In a total community survey in South Africa, when they took blacks and whites relative to their numbers in the community, it was amazing—they found sixteen times as many centenarians amongst the blacks as amongst the whites. Lots of people think you don't get old blacks. There are lots of old blacks. Those who are 45 or 50 have a statistically better chance of getting to eighty than white people have. They're not going to die of coronary heart disease or lung cancer or bowel cancer or these things."

So while an American is more likely to survive infancy, he or she is far more likely to be killed by the diseases of midlife. And the reason is diet. "All of these diseases really are manifestations of maladaptation to a new environment," Burkitt said. "Western man has made more change in his diet over the last six or eight generations—150 to 200 years—than man has made throughout the whole of his sojourn on earth. We have suddenly plunged into an environment to which we are not adapted. Our bodies are the same as Stone Age bodies genetically, anatomically, physiologically, and everything else. But what we put into them is quite different. We are putting supermarket food into Stone Age bodies. In lectures I often use a picture of a Stone Age man with a club over his shoulder pushing a trolley into a supermarket. We're not adapted. It's no good saying let's wait until we adapt because that might take another ten thousand years. The only thing we can do is to go back a bit."

> *"Western man has made more change in his diet over the last six or eight generations-150 to 200 years-than man has made throughout the whole of his sojourn on earth."*
>
> **Dr. Denis Burkitt**

We need to bring back the fiber—that is, unrefined plant foods, particularly grains and legumes. We also need to cut back on the meats, dairy products, and fried foods—the high-fat fare, devoid of fiber and carbohydrate, that has insinuated its way into our diet.

"I first thought fiber was almost the whole thing," Burkitt said. "Now I recognize it's a question of fiber, starch, fat, salt, and sugar. They all play a role. Cleave would never accept that fat played a role, and he died of atherosclerosis himself a few years ago."

Constipation

The refining of grains has led, over the last two centuries, to the gradual disappearance of fiber from the diet. Whole wheat bread has been replaced by soft white bread. Other whole grains find no place in the diet of modern Western countries. In the digestive tract, fiber holds water, which keeps the intestinal contents soft. Without fiber to hold water, digestion compacts the intestinal contents, which then move only very slowly. As a result, constipation has become almost a routine in the modern world.

"It has been said very authoritatively that if we got the fiber back in our diet, the whole of the laxative industry would be in liquidation within six months," Burkitt said. "Because fiber holds water. The only reason you have a laxative industry is because you've taken fiber out of your diet. And I mean cereal fiber. Never kid yourself that you're getting much fiber by eating salad. Americans eat more salad than any nation on Earth, and they're the most constipated nation on the globe. So it doesn't help them at all. It's got to be cereal fiber. Beans are also good. Cabbage might help you a little bit, but fruit and green vegetables by and large are not much help from the point of view of constipation.

> *"The only reason you have a laxative industry is because you've taken fiber out of your diet."*
>
> **Dr. Denis Burkitt**

"Until a hundred years ago there was no cold storage and no canning. There was no way of storing food. The human race was adapted to live on what you could store on the floor of the barn. Those were cereals, whether it be wheat, rye, or others;

legumes: peas and beans; millets and tubers: potatoes, carrots, turnips, and so on. Those are the things which we are no longer eating. We've thrown out our potatoes, and we've thrown out our bread."

The cure for constipation? Whole grains, such as wheat, oatmeal, and brown rice, and beans and other legumes in generous portions. When these are part of the daily diet, regularity follows.

Varicose Veins, Hemorrhoids, and Hiatus Hernia

As a result of the constipation that occurs on a fiber-depleted diet, straining to pass stools is a daily occurrence. Over the long run, this daily battle with constipation leads to other problems. The increase in pressure in the abdomen caused by straining is implicated as a cause of varicose veins, hemorrhoids, and hiatal hernia, as Burkitt explains:

"When you strain at stool, you put very high pressures in your abdominal cavity," Burkitt said. "These pressures are immediately transmitted to the veins draining the lower limbs. The pressures are held back at the first set of valves in the leg veins. Now it has been shown that the valves in the leg give way sequentially one after the other from above down. When all the valves are incompetent, gravity plus straining can make pressures in the veins of the lower part of the leg nearly as high as the blood pressures in arteries."

> *"Never kid yourself that you're getting much fiber by eating salad. Americans eat more salad than any nation on Earth, and they're the most constipated nation on the globe."*
>
> **Dr. Denis Burkitt**

Under these pressures, veins are damaged. Varicose veins can result. Other evidence also indicates that abdominal straining can cause varicose veins. "People in Southeast Asia who ride tri-shaws struggle along with a couple of people sitting in front. They have far more varicose veins than people who stand all day cutting hair. People who climb the Himalayas carrying heavy loads tend to get varicose veins. Now these are consistent with straining as one cause." They are straining the abdomen and pushing blood down into the veins of the leg. Straining to pass stools does precisely the same thing.

Burkitt hypothesizes that hemorrhoids are caused by the same mechanism. Hemorrhoids are engorgements of normal blood vessels. Just as the veins of the legs distend under pressure, the hemorrhoidal vessels do the same thing. Repeated straining of the abdomen to pass stools forces blood to engorge the hemorrhoidal vessels. The solution is to make stools easier to pass. This is where fiber works: It retains water so that stools pass easily. Constipation is prevented and straining is unnecessary.

Increased pressures in the abdomen may also contribute to hiatus (or hiatal) hernia. Hiatus hernia is a condition in which part of the stomach is pushed upward through the diaphragm into the chest cavity. It typically causes no symptoms, but may contribute to heartburn for some patients.

"My hypothesis for hiatus hernia is beginning to be accepted by gastroenterologists," Burkitt said. "If you take a tennis ball and cut a hole in it and fill it with water and squeeze the tennis ball, the water goes out through the hole. Now, your abdominal cavity is the tennis ball. And every time you squeeze your tennis ball to void constipated stools you force the stomach out through the hole in the diaphragm which transmits the esophagus. Now, we have never found any community in the world which passes large soft stools and gets hiatus hernia."

For these conditions, medical teaching has often ignored the causative role of dietary factors. "If you look in a textbook it will say that varicose veins are due to pregnancies or large abdominal tumors or standing. That's rubbish. It's just totally denied by the evidence," Burkitt said. "Total community surveys in North America have shown 50 percent of women over the age of 40 to have varicose veins. A recent study in New Guinea found only one varicose vein amongst 800 adult women. So how can you say that varicose veins are due to man not being adapted to the upright posture? We've had many surveys done in Africa and India. Most of them were under five percent.

"If you looked up the cause of hiatus hernia in our most popular surgical textbooks, it is said to be due to the lack of tone in the diaphragm with advancing age. But why is it that the diaphragm never lacks tone in Africa or India or the Middle East or Japan and only does in North America and Western Europe? This doesn't tell you anything, does it? Then it tells you it's due to large abdominal tumors, but a country with large abdominal tumors gets no hiatus hernia. Thirdly, it suggests it's due to pregnancy, when the countries with the most pregnancies have the least hiatus hernia. Fourthly, in an edition in the mid-1970s, it said 'women wearing corsets.' Well, how many women wear corsets?

"Again, if you have hypotheses which are totally at variance with evidence, you've got to scrap them, haven't you? I wrote this up in the *American Journal of Clinical Nutrition,* and they gave it an editorial. The whole editorial gave reasons why it must be wrong. In the last paragraph, the fellow writing the editorial said, 'Nevertheless if I was a betting man I'd bet Burkitt was right.' So that was encouraging."

Appendicitis

Appendicitis is rare in countries that have a high-fiber diet, according to numerous epidemiologic studies. In Uganda, Burkitt noticed that the only Africans who tended to develop appendicitis were those who had adopted Western dietary habits. He became wary about diagnosing appendicitis in Africans unless they could speak English, indicating their degree of contact with Western culture.

The appendix is a small, finger-like tube attached to the large intestine. It can become blocked by a small, compacted lump of stool. This blockage can lead to inflammation and infection, and characteristic abdominal pain. Removal of the appendix is then usually necessary.

Burkitt hypothesizes that the reason appendicitis is rare in countries maintaining traditional diets is that the fiber in their diet keeps stools soft, and so the appendix does not become blocked. If Westerners were to return the fiber to their diets, this common surgical emergency might become a medical rarity.

Fiber, Cholesterol, and Gallstones

Fiber helps lower cholesterol. Evidence shows that this is especially true of soluble fiber, such as oat bran. While this effect is partly due to the fact that high-fiber foods tend to displace high-fat foods from the menu, there may be other mechanisms involved. In the liver, cholesterol is turned into bile acids which are sent into the intestinal tract where they help in digestion. These bile acids can be reabsorbed and returned to the body's cholesterol pool. But fiber can trap bile acids in the intestinal tract and allow them to be excreted. This helps lower the cholesterol level in the blood.

This is obviously important in the prevention of heart disease. But there is another important benefit too: preventing gallstones. Cholesterol can form stones in the gallbladder. These stones can be the cause of persistent abdominal pain, and often lead to surgery. Removal of the gallbladder has become one of the commonest abdominal operations.

"There's a lot of evidence coming out now that fiber is protective against gallstones," Burkitt said. "If you feed volunteers high-fiber diets, you lower their cholesterol, and the bile has less of a tendency to form stones."

In addition, a high-fiber diet appears to increase the formation of a particular bile acid, called *chenodeoxycholate*, which has gallstone-dissolving properties. In combination with fiber's cholesterol-lowering effect, gallstones are much less likely to form.

"The great thing is we don't need to know these mechanisms in order to take action," Burkitt said. "It doesn't really matter what the mechanism is as long as you can demonstrate that a certain thing gives you the right results."

In America, gallbladder operations are an everyday event. In countries with a low-fat, high-fiber diet, they are rarely necessary. It is only those who adopt the diet of affluent countries who are at significant risk for the disease. "I only removed two gallbladders from Africans in my twenty years in Africa," Burkitt said. "One was a queen, one of the only two queens I ever operated on. So fifty percent of my gallstones were taken out of queens."

How much fiber should we actually be getting in our diet? "At the moment we are getting about twenty grams a day, in some parts of England only ten and some parts of America only ten. We ought to have a minimum of thirty grams, preferably forty, and it ought to be cereal fiber in particular. If we did only one thing in this country, if we multiplied our bread intake by two or three and never had it made from white flour, that would revolutionize the health of America."

The key factor, of course, is not to count the number of grams of fiber consumed each day, but rather to shift the diet so that healthy amounts of fiber, fat, and protein naturally fall into place. This means a new emphasis on grains, legumes, vegetables, and fruits. As we do this, we will look better, feel better, and live free of many of the common problems that could otherwise take away the enjoyment of life.

Diabetes

In diabetes, the cells of the body cannot get the sugar they need. Glucose, a simple sugar, is the body's main fuel. It is present in the blood, but in diabetics it cannot get into the cells where it is needed. When diabetes starts in childhood, it is due to an inadequate supply of insulin, the hormone which ushers sugar into the cells of the body. Without insulin, the cell membranes keep sugar out. When diabetes begins in adulthood, it is not due to an inadequate supply of insulin. There is plenty of insulin in the blood stream, but the cells do not respond readily to it. Sugar cannot get into the cells, and it backs up in the blood stream. In the short run, diabetics may experience episodes of labored breathing, vomiting, and dehydration. In the long run, diabetics are at risk for heart disease, kidney problems, disorders of vision, and other difficulties.

The dietary approach to diabetes is illustrated by a treatment program that has been very helpful for people with the disease, called the Pritikin Program. The foundation of the program is not the ever-increasing regimen of medicines that has been the mainstay against diabetes over the last several decades, but, rather, replacing medicines as much as possible with low-fat foods and exercise.

Monroe Rosenthal, M.D., is the Medical Director of the Pritikin Program. Rosenthal is lean and athletic. When he is not working with patients to reverse the damage of years of bad diet at the Pritikin Center on the ocean front in Santa Monica, California, he can be found running marathons. He explains his approach to diabetes, "In the mid to late seventies, a popular belief was that since sugar is found in the urine of diabetics, that by not eating sugar or substances that are turned into sugar, such as starches, breads, fruit, and so forth, they would improve. This was really a misconception. When you take away the complex carbohydrates and refined sugars from the diet you're left with fat and protein."

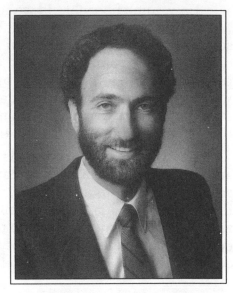

Dr. Monroe Rosenthal

Fat, in particular, is a problem for diabetics. The more fat there is in the diet, the harder time insulin has in getting sugar into the cell. Exactly how fat disables insulin's action is not clear. But what is clear is that minimizing fat helps insulin do its job much better. "By switching to a lower-fat diet," Rosenthal said, "whatever insulin is available seems to work more effectively at incorporating sugar into the cells."

To reduce fat in the diet, the program drastically reduces meats, high-fat dairy products, and oils. At the same time, it increases grains, legumes, and vegetables. One study found that 21 of 23 patients on oral medications and 13 of 17 patients on insulin were able to get off their medication after 26 days on the program.[2] At two- and three-year follow-ups, most diabetics treated with this regimen have retained their gains.[3] The dietary changes are simple, but profound, and they work.

But there is a second essential component to managing diabetes. Through regular exercise, the need for insulin injections can often be reduced, and oral medications often become unnecessary. "An aerobic exercise program will allow sugar to enter the cells without the use of insulin," Rosenthal said. "This holds true not only for the adult patients but also to some extent for insulin-dependent juvenile diabetics. Exercising muscles have a voracious appetite for fuel. When an individual is engaged in regular aerobic exercise, the sugar is able to enter the cells without the need for as much, or any, insulin. The cells just sort of suck up the circulating sugar.

"We see many individuals who are on insulin because they're overweight, not exercising, and eating a lot of refined sugar and fat. Through diet and regular aerobic exercise, we can essentially get them off insulin and off oral agents, and get them to normal blood sugar values."

The Pritikin Diet limits fat to no more than ten percent of daily calories. The diet and exercise regimen is so potent that if medicines are not reduced, the blood sugar lowering may be too strong. "We take all individuals off oral agents when they come in," Rosenthal said. "That's not to say that some don't go back on. But the effects of the diet and exercise program are so potent that if we don't discontinue oral medication, a very large percentage will wind up with a hypoglycemic reaction within the first couple days. For those on insulin, we cut back about a third of their insulin right away to avoid getting into problems with hypoglycemic episodes. So the program itself is quite potent when you combine the aerobic exercise with the lack of refined sugar, lack of alcohol, and lack of fat in the diet."

While people with adult-onset diabetes can often eliminate medications when their weight is reduced and foods and exercise are better controlled, those with childhood-onset diabetes will always need a source of insulin. The causes of insulin-dependent (childhood-onset) diabetes remain elusive. Although genetic factors may be responsible for a predisposition to diabetes, it may be that other factors, such as nutrition, determine whether diabetes actually develops. Recent studies have implicated milk consumption as a contributor.[4] When milk consumption patterns were examined across various countries, there was a very strong correlation with the incidence of insulin-dependent diabetes. Studies of diabetic patients suggest that milk proteins cause an autoimmune reaction in which the body mistakenly attacks its own insulin-producing cells.[5] Even so, a good diet and regular exercise can minimize the amount of insulin these diabetics require. This is especially important given their tendency toward complications. Heart disease and other blood vessel problems are much more common in diabetics. So it is doubly important to keep fit and to keep fats in the diet to a minimum.

Rosenthal feels that diabetics are short-changed by the diets most doctors give them. "The typical American Diabetes Association diet is a diet high in fat. They limit the amount of butter, they cut down on eggs and so forth, but it still contains about 300 milligrams of cholesterol per day and around 30 percent fat. It's approaching our diet at a very tediously slow pace."

This book is not intended as a comprehensive program for diabetes. If you have diabetes, you will need to work with your doctor in a program tailored for your needs. But it is important to recognize that diabetes is a disease that, for many, need never occur. And for most who have it, it can be much more manageable with a food plan that gets most of its calories from complex carbohydrates while minimizing fats. At the same time, regular vigorous exercise helps insulin to work optimally.

Problems with Protein: Osteoporosis & Kidney Damage

Osteoporosis—the loss of bone tissue—is common in Western countries, particularly in women after menopause. Changes in diet and life-style may help prevent it. The key is not in milk or massive calcium supplements. Advertisements by the dairy industry notwithstanding, evidence shows that, beyond a certain minimum, eating calcium does little to help the body build bones.

"We have no evidence that osteoporosis has anything to do with calcium intake," Burkitt said, "and there is very great doubt as to whether giving calcium has any effect on osteoporosis." *Science* magazine on August 1, 1986, noted "the large body of evidence indicating no relationship between calcium intake and bone density." Dr. B. Lawrence Riggs of the

Mayo Clinic measured bone densities and calcium intake in women for several years. He reported, "We found no correlation at all between calcium intake and bone loss, not even a trend." Some studies have found an effect of calcium intake on the density of the wrist bones, but little or no effect where it counts—the spine and hip.

What causes osteoporosis? First of all, hormones play a major role. After menopause, hormonal changes foster the loss of bone. Doctors often prescribe hormone supplements to women for precisely this reason. Such treatments are helpful in delaying osteoporosis, although their overall health risk remains controversial. But this is only part of the story. Another major factor appears to be the damaging effect of a high-protein diet.[6-9]

"The literature indicates that a high-protein diet, which the American diet certainly is, contributes to the epidemic of osteoporosis," Rosenthal said. "We have a population that eats a high-protein diet, they don't exercise much, they smoke. Those are really the main reasons for the epidemic of osteoporosis."

An overly generous amount of protein in the diet depletes the body's calcium. When protein is taken in, some is used for the body's various needs. Some of the excess is changed to urea in the liver. Urea is a powerful diuretic. When urea and the amino acids, which are the building blocks of proteins, enter the kidneys, they cause the loss of water and the loss of important minerals as well. Calcium is one of the minerals that is washed away in this process. In addition, as proteins break down to amino acids which are absorbed into the blood stream, the blood becomes slightly more acidic. To neutralize this acidic effect, calcium is pulled from bone material. This ultimately leads to an increase in calcium

> *"We have no evidence that osteoporosis has anything to do with calcuim intake, and there is very great doubt as to whether giving calcium has any effect on osteoporosis."*
>
> **Dr. Denis Burkitt**

excretion in the urine. So the more protein we take in beyond the amount we need, the more calcium we lose.

"Researchers have estimated that doubling the protein in the diet leads to a 50 percent increase in calcium loss in the urine," says physician and nutrition author John A. McDougall, M.D. Like the Pritikin Center, McDougall has found that dietary changes can be phenomenally success- ful in treating a variety of illnesses. He sees pa- tients at the St. Helena Hospital in Deer Park, California, and appears

> *"We have a population that eats a high-protein diet, they don't exercise much, they smoke. Those are really the main rea- sons for the epidemic of osteoporosis."*
>
> **Dr. Monroe Rosenthal**

frequently on radio and television programs. He is concerned about osteoporosis and the failure of most doctors to address its causes. Calcium supplements simply do not eliminate the loss of calcium caused by a high-protein diet.

"Calcium supplements are usually ineffective in com- pensating for this loss," McDougall said. "Studies of Eskimo populations have shown that their tremendous intake of fish protein is accompanied by significant osteoporosis. Eskimos over the age of 40 have an average of 10 to 15 percent less bone tissue than do comparable Caucasians in the U.S. The Eskimo diet includes a large quantity of fish bones, so they have a very high calcium intake, as high as 2500 milligrams a day. The damage done by their high-protein diet is not compensated for by all the calcium they consume."

Americans get into trouble not only with the amount of protein they eat but with the *type* of protein as well. "There are about 20 common amino acids that make up the dif- ferent proteins," McDougall said. "Three of these contain the element sulfur in their chemical structure. These sulfur- containing amino acids have a strong calcium-depleting effect on the kidneys. Animal proteins have a higher content of these sulfur-containing amino acids than do vegetable proteins."

Meats, including poultry and fish, contain too much protein and too high a concentration of the sulfur-containing amino acids. But there is new evidence of another problem with meats: they are very poor sources of boron, which appears to be important in preventing osteoporosis, according to research conducted by Dr. Forrest H. Nielsen, a research nutritionist with the U.S. Department of Agriculture.[10,11] "The best way to get boron," Dr. Nielsen writes, "is through a balanced diet containing an abundance of fruits, vegetables, nuts, and legumes." Milk is very low in the element, and meat and eggs have no detectable boron. Boron appears to help stop the loss of calcium from the body, and adjusts the levels of sex hormones which affect bone metabolism. The data on boron, however, is new, and is being explored in further studies.

> *"Reserachers have estimated that doubling the protein in the diet leads to a 50 percent increase in clacium loss in the urine."*
>
> *Dr. John McDougall*

Some have suggested that a high-fiber diet may reduce our ability to absorb calcium. The phytic acid in the grains supposedly binds calcium and prevents its absorption from the digestive tract. Burkitt disagrees. "That's absolute baloney. Phytic acid does bind calcium, but the evidence that phytic acid in cereals prejudices your calcium levels is only valid in short-term experiments in rodents. It has never been shown to be valid in long-term experiments in man. You very quickly adapt. There have been large studies showing that a high-fiber diet doesn't prejudice your mineral metabolism."

Burkitt cites the work of Alec Walker, showing that populations eating little meat and a great deal of fiber had very little osteoporosis. "Africans have a much lower calcium intake than we do with a three times larger fiber intake, and they suffer far less from demineralization of the skeleton. He's tested all this by X-raying the bones. Age-adjusted, Africans get about a tenth as many femoral neck fractures when they get old as people in America do."*

To prevent osteoporosis, we must also *use* our bones. Weight-bearing exercise helps build strong bones. In addition, we need to be aware that alcohol and tobacco aggravate

---

*The femoral neck is part of the thigh bone at the hip.

bone loss. And keeping our protein intake to more modest levels is important.

The dairy industry, of course, is using osteoporosis as a marketing tool. They would like us to believe that the body's careful regulation of calcium absorption and bone structure can be tricked by simply ingesting a large amount of milk. "But it's not valid," Burkitt said. "People with quite low calcium intake get infinitely less osteoporosis."

McDougall adds another reason to avoid dairy products: the milk proteins often elicit allergic responses. "Dairy products are the most common cause of food allergies," McDougall said. "Look at all the allergic reactions to dairy products that have been noted in the scientific literature: canker sores, digestive problems, skin conditions, respiratory reactions, and so on." This is a separate problem from lactose intolerance, the inability to digest the milk sugar, which causes indigestion in many Africans and Asians. Dairy allergy is a sensitivity to the milk proteins, and is often manifested in subtle ways, as McDougall points out, "People don't know until they get away from them for a while, and then try them again. And they say, 'Oh, that's why I had a stuffy nose all the time,' or 'That's why I have post-nasal drip.' That's why I try to get my patients to change completely. When people avoid dairy products completely, they often find improvement in symptoms which they did not realize were caused by milk proteins."

Milk consumption is also implicated as a contributor to cataracts. Although there are other factors, such as excessive exposure to sunlight, which contribute to opacities of the lens, it has been suggested that *galactose*, a breakdown product of the milk sugar *lactose*, may gradually damage the lens. Indeed, a detailed review of the subject published in 1982 showed that populations which consume large amounts of dairy products tend to have a much higher incidence of cataracts than populations which avoid dairy products.[12] Nursing children are better able to break down both lactose and galactose. But as children grow older, the capacity to metabolize these compounds diminishes. Many Caucasian adults can break down lactose well, but do not rapidly metabolize the galactose which comes from it. As a result, they are at risk for the problems which may be caused by high levels of galactose.

The correlation between the use of dairy products and cataracts is real, but the cause-and-effect relationship is only theoretical, awaiting more observation. In Chapter 3, the link between milk consumption and ovarian cancer was discussed.

This does not mean that we do not need calcium in the diet. We do. There are sources of calcium which do not create the problems dairy products do. Green vegetables, such as broccoli, collard greens, and kale, are loaded with calcium. Fortified orange juice and many common varieties of beans are also rich in calcium. The key is to insure that these foods are included in the diet, while also reducing the loss of calcium from the body by limiting protein intake to reasonable amounts.

> *"Dairy products are the most common cause of food allergies. When people avoid dairy products completely, they often find improvement in symptoms which they did not realize were caused by milk proteins."*
>
> **Dr. John McDougall**

Excess protein is related to more than osteoporosis. It also leads to kidney damage. This is of particular concern for those who already have suffered some loss of kidney function, and doctors will generally advise these patients to limit their protein intake. People who have a history of kidney infections, or have donated a kidney, or have diabetes, atherosclerosis, or high blood pressure will also want to protect their kidneys. That means limiting protein intake. Evidence suggests that excessive protein causes a gradual decline in kidney function for those who are otherwise healthy.[13-15]

The average American diet contains far more protein than our bodies really need. It can't be stored in the body the way excess calories are stored as body fat. The breakdown products of proteins are filtered out by the kidneys. In the process, these breakdown products raise fluid pressures in the nephrons, which are the filter units of the kidney. The nephrons are over-worked. This process appears to speed up the destruction of kidney tissue.

As the problems with osteoporosis and kidney disease indicate, it is important not to overdo it on protein.

Sexual Functioning

Not long ago, I was giving a lecture in Lubbock, Texas. As I spelled out the evidence on how a bad diet leads to heart disease and strokes, a group of students in the back of the room began to mutter and complain. They were studying beef and pork production and were not about to hear criticisms of the agriculture industry. I described the process of atherosclerosis, commonly known as "hardening of the arteries," which chokes off the blood supply to the heart muscle, causing heart attacks and often death. The same process occurs in the arteries to the brain, leading to strokes—the death of a portion of the brain. Howls of laughter came from the back of the room, sprinkled with heckling. They did not want to believe the message.

"You can laugh all you want," I said. "But this process of atherosclerosis doesn't just cause heart attacks. It also causes *impotence*." Total silence fell on the room. Suddenly, we were not discussing the remote afflictions of middle age. The very essence of masculinity was threatened.

Can diet be related to impotence? The answer is yes. A study of 440 impotent men was published in the *Lancet* in January, 1985.[16] The risk factors that have been identified for heart disease were present in the impotent men far more commonly than in the general population (See Chapter 1). Just as a loss of blood flow to the heart muscle leads to the death of a portion of the heart, the loss of blood flow to the genitals interferes with sexual potency. Ultimately, impotence can result. The study concluded that "the increase in the frequency of impotence with age is mainly related to arteriosclerotic changes . . . ." The high-fat, high-cholesterol diet is a principal culprit.

But the connections between diet and impotence do not end there. As we noted in this chapter, diet contributes to diabetes. In turn, diabetes often leads to impotence, both because atherosclerosis is more aggressive in diabetics and because gradual damage to peripheral nerves also occurs in many diabetics. Above, we reviewed some basics of the dietary control of diabetes.

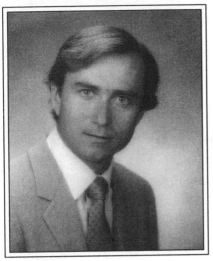

Dr. John McDougall

Diet is also an important factor in hypertension, which also contributes to impotence by way of its effect on atherosclerosis. In addition, some of the medications used in the treatment of hypertension can interfere with sexual functioning. Methyldopa (Aldomet) frequently leads to impotence. Guanethidine commonly causes inhibition of ejaculation. Ironically, although high blood pressure can be a very serious condition, it often has no symptoms that the patient can feel. So when men are treated with drugs which cause impotence, they may find they have little motivation to take the drugs as prescribed. Because hypertension is a serious condition, however, any change in medications should be discussed with your doctor. In Chapter 1, we looked at how a high-fat diet can lead to high blood pressure and how a lower-fat diet, particularly a vegetarian diet, can lower blood pressure. Some people will continue to need medications, but many can use a dietary approach instead.

McDougall strongly encourages giving the dietary approach a try. "Many men on blood pressure pills are impotent," McDougall said. "I'll ask if they'd like to try beans and rice instead." In his years of practice in Hawaii, McDougall consistently noticed that Asian men on traditional diets which omitted dairy products and contained relatively little meat not only lived longer, they also remained sexually functional throughout their lives. "Sometimes men would start new families when they were 70 years old," McDougall said. "They could function sexually at 70 years old. And they were going to see their children grow up and go to high school and so on. They didn't plan on dying at 72. They planned to live to be 85 or 90, and so they did, and in good health."

The sexual function of women is affected also. As we saw in Chapter 3, a high-fat diet artificially elevates the amounts of estrogens in the blood stream and is implicated in the progressive reduction in the age of puberty in women. In addition, the milk sugar, lactose, has also been implicated in damage to ovary function and even linked to cancer of the ovary. Further research is needed to elucidate these relationships between diet and the sex hormones of women.

Denis Burkitt on the Role of Medicine

In his pioneering research on cancer, and, more recently, on nutrition, Denis Burkitt's methods were as unique as his findings. Burkitt solved his medical questions, not with test tubes and laboratory equipment mainly, but by carefully studying populations. For the most part, the information he needed was not readily available. So he went out and got it. He spent a tremendous amount of time traveling around Africa and much of the rest of the world, including places beyond the reach of roads, to see the places which were struck by disease and those which were not. Then he analyzed his data to see what he could find.

Initially, he discovered, and cured, Burkitt's lymphoma. He then took on a much bigger target in trying to reform the dietary habits of Western countries. But he also recognized the need to redirect medical research and practice.

"First of all, medical students ought to have in their curriculum a course on nutrition and not waste their time learning about cancer surgery or heart surgery until later in their specialist careers," Burkitt said.

"When I worked for twelve years at the Medical Research Council, my senior used to adjudicate all applications for grants. He wrote two words at the end of every request: 'So what?' Now if all research grants had 'So what?' written at the end of them, you'd cut them down by about three-quarters. An awful lot of them have no practical application. And in this stage of life, we ought to be looking for practical applications."

Is Burkitt suggesting that much of the research going on nowadays isn't really worth a whole lot? "Absolute waste of money. And there is one other thing. The National Cancer Institute asked me to lecture there. I started my lecture by saying I thought the biggest defect in cancer research today was specializing in cancer, which must have shaken them a bit. If you try to find out the cause of a disease like bowel cancer, you've got to look at all the other diseases associated with it. You see, I get credited for the idea that fiber might be protective against bowel cancer, but I got into that by recognizing that you never get diverticular disease in a community that hasn't got a high rate of bowel cancer.* They go together. Now, you forget about the cancer; you look at the diverticular disease, and you find that diverticular disease is related to low-fiber diets. Couldn't cancer be the same? But the cancer specialist seldom looks at anything except cancer. He doesn't even record polyps in his registry. And since colon cancer is nearly always derived from polyps in America, and there are a hundred or a thousand times as many polyps as cancers, why not get rid of cancer research altogether and look for the cause of polyps? Then you've got the answer."

Burkitt is not saying that research has not given us benefits. "It's given us enormous benefits, but all the really major advances in medicine have been in the realm of preventing disease rather than in the realm of cure. Look at poliomyelitis which, when I was a student, was crippling all over. Diphtheria is gone. Tuberculosis is gone. And smallpox is gone, the biggest advance in this century. All the major advances of medicine are in the field of prevention. Now, I wouldn't be allowed to say this unless I spent thirty years on the curative side. But now that I'm older, I'm allowed to say it. You can't challenge that. Nobody can challenge it.

"We got rid of infective disease by increasing resistance and by getting rid of the causes—clean water, clean milk, adequate sewage disposal, and so on. Doctors and drugs had nothing whatever to do with the conquest of infective disease. If you look at the mortality rates from an infective disease in Britain between 1850 and the second World War, they had almost reached their present levels before the sulfonamides and antibiotics were invented. The general concept that doc-

---

Diverticulosis is a condition in which pouches form in the wall of the large intestine (colon). When these pouches become inflamed, the condition is known as diverticulitis.

tors and drugs affect the health of a community is rubbish. Doctors and drugs have no effect on the health of a community. They have a profound effect on sick people, but not on the health of a community.

"If you take even tuberculosis, when streptomycin and PAS came in, the mid-19th century figures of pulmonary tuberculosis had already fallen by 94 percent. When we got these wonderful drugs they were marvelous. They halved the mortality rate. But that was from six to three. They went from one hundred to six with no drugs at all."

Burkitt gave another example of the strength of preventive measures: the control of cholera. The case illustrates how the cause of disease has to be removed, whether or not we have a full understanding of how it actually produces the disease. "A man called Snow investigated a cholera epidemic in London. He was an anesthetist. He found that all the people suffering from cholera in that area got their water from the same pump in Broad Street.

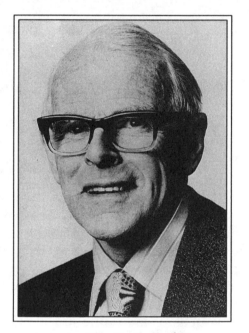

Dr. Denis Burkitt

He asked the local councilors if he could have permission to take the handle off the pump. They all thought he was mad. But he did that, and the cholera epidemic subsided, because the pump drew the water from the Thames below the site where the sewage was emitted. They discovered, therefore, that cholera was related to sewage-contaminated water. But it wasn't until twenty-five years later that the *Vibrio cholera* organism was identified. You didn't have to identify the organism before removing the cause of cholera. You've got to recognize the cause and remove it, but you don't have to understand it.

"Percival Pott recognized that scrotal cancer was due to people sweeping chimneys. He was able to persuade people not to let little children sweep chimneys, and they didn't get scrotal cancer. But it wasn't until half a century later that hydrocarbons were recognized as a cause of cancer. We don't have to know all the details before we can take action.

"I was in Cincinnati some years ago, and after my lecture a man came to speak to me. He told me that he was chosen by the government to advise people on diet and health. He said, 'I understand what you're talking about, but I'm not going to advise anybody until I understand all the mechanisms and have double-blind trials, and what have you.' 'Well,' I said, 'Diverticular disease is going to take a sixty-year trial, so it'll be your grandson writing up the last paper. If you were on a pier and your son fell into the water, I know what you'd do. If you had a life jacket in your hand, you wouldn't throw it to him. You'd say, "I'm not quite sure of the specific gravity of this life jacket, and I don't really know whether it fits my son. I think I'll go back to the lab. I'll do three more weeks' work on my life jacket, then I'll come back to the harbor and, if Jimmy's still swimming around, I'll throw him the life jacket" But we don't work that way. This is armchair science.

"Fiber is something which we didn't understand, didn't know how to measure, and didn't know what it did until less than twenty years ago. So we said, 'Let's take it out.' We didn't understand tonsils until we discovered T-cells and B-cells in the early 1960s. What did we do with tonsils? Took them out. We didn't understand the appendix—chop it out. There have been several papers now showing that if you have had your tonsils and your appendix out, you've got a bigger chance of getting certain cancers, notably Hodgkins' Disease, than if you keep them. We didn't understand hemorrhoids—nip 'em off. But this is the kind of arrogant approach to medicine: if you don't understand something, you cut it out. And now we recognize that you can't do that. God didn't give us any of these things just for fun."

Chapter 7

Foods and the Mind

"One cannot think well, love well, sleep well,
if one has not dined well."
Virginia Woolf

Foods affect the brain in many ways. Some foods make us sleep. Others help us stay alert. Sugar can have either positive or negative effects, depending on what else is part of the meal. Alcohol, likewise, can be a sedative or a stimulant, depending on timing and genetics. Even NutraSweet can affect brain chemistry. Foods can affect a child's performance in school and even the basic functioning of the child's brain.

Over the short-term and the long-term, brain function is adjusted by the contents of the dinner plate. Some food ingredients affect the brain directly. Certain mushrooms, for example, have a potent hallucinogenic effect. Nutmeg has also been used as a recreational drug. Although small amounts of the spice have no discernible effect, the ingestion of two grated nutmegs causes, after several hours, feelings of unreality and the sense that one is out of one's body. The arms and legs feel like lead. Fear and agitation, dry mouth, thirst, rapid pulse, and a flushing of the face can also occur.[1] Likewise, caffeine has predictable effects on the brain. Under its influence, thought is clearer and more rapid. Reaction time is quicker. There is an increased sensitivity to the environment.

But caffeine is habituating. Withdrawal causes headaches and fatigue. Among the other negative effects of caffeine are tremulousness, anxiety, and loss of calcium from the body. Caffeine is found in coffee, of course, but also in tea, cocoa, cola drinks, and numerous over-the-counter pain relievers and stimulants. Other foods allow us to actually manipulate certain brain chemicals called neurotransmitters, which are important in alertness, sleep, depression, and mental acuity. But first, let us take a detailed look at two parts of the diet that can have profound effects on the brain. One, alcohol, is older than history. The other, NutraSweet, is the latest of the massively popular chemical additives.

Alcohol

Alcohol is a universal sedative. Under its influence, anxieties melt away and inhibitions dissolve. We find ourselves talking, laughing, singing, or doing other things we would normally do with more restraint.

As soon as alcohol arrives in the stomach, it begins to be absorbed. Within minutes it arrives in the brain, where it works on the cell membranes of each individual brain cell. These cells use their membranes in order to communicate with each other. Under alcohol's influence, the membranes expand and become distorted.[2] They begin to have trouble getting messages to and from each other, and a feeling of intoxication develops.

Alcohol definitely does reduce anxiety. It affects the same part of the brain cells that is affected by Valium (diazapam) and other anxiety-reducing drugs. Like Valium, alcohol's anti-anxiety effect lasts beyond the period when alcohol is in the blood. Intoxication may have passed, but brain effects continue. The anxiety-reducing effect of alcohol has even been used as a medical treatment. In an unusual study, researchers offered psychiatric patients an hour each day in a hospital "pub," complete with music, television, checkered tablecloths, and beer. The combination of alcohol and social interaction helped reduce psychiatric symptoms.[3]

On the other hand, the chronic effects of alcohol cause psychiatric disorders and mimic others in millions of people.

Regular alcohol use can lead to depression that is indistinguishable from depression caused by other factors. In alcohol dependency, withdrawal can cause hallucinations, seizures, and even death. Chronic heavy alcohol consumption leads to a serious loss of mental faculties.

Over the short term, the brain tries to fight back. The brain cell membranes adjust to counteract alcohol's effects. You may have noticed this effect if you have had several drinks during an evening. The initial drinks have the greatest effect, but the brain cells adapt somewhat and diminish the effect of subsequent drinks.

Alcohol's Dr. Jekyll and Acetaldehyde

Some of alcohol's effects are not due to the alcohol itself, but to its first cousin, *acetaldehyde*. This compound is naturally produced from alcohol as the alcohol molecule is broken down in the body. Acetaldehyde is, in turn, broken down and excreted. But if acetaldehyde is made from alcohol faster than it can be removed, it builds up in the blood stream. Unlike alcohol, whose effects are usually experienced as pleasant, acetaldehyde may cause very unpleasant effects. If acetaldehyde builds up, it causes a flushed appearance, headache, nausea and vomiting, rapid pulse, and low blood pressure.[4]

A glass of wine or other alcohol promotes sleep. But acetaldehyde is stimulating and may cause early morning awakening. For some people, particularly women, rather little acetaldehyde accumulates; for others, the amounts are quite significant. So while alcohol may promote sleep, one might find oneself wide awake before dawn, unable to return to sleep.

Genetic factors play a role. Many Asians break down acetaldehyde only very slowly. When they have a drink, it builds up in the blood causing the unpleasant flushing reaction and a distaste for alcohol ever after. Everyone's tendency to build up this toxic product is different and is largely genetically determined. Those who build up large amounts of acetaldehyde have a very different experience with alcohol than those who do not. Our patterns of alcohol use, including the risk for alcoholism, are partly determined by these genetic factors.

Aspartame: Brain Effects of NutraSweet®

NutraSweet has taken the diet food industry by storm. Research shows, however, that the chemical sweetener may be inadvertently causing a storm of a different sort: a storm inside our brain cells. Aspartame, the chemical marketed as NutraSweet, is a combination of two amino acids—phenylalanine and aspartic acid. Richard Wurtman, M.D., a researcher at the Massachusetts Institute of Technology in Cambridge, Massachusetts, found that the chemical may promote convulsions. He published in the medical journal, *The Lancet,* reports of three people who had had grand mal seizures, collapsing as their muscles jerked violently, after consuming large amounts of NutraSweet-flavored soft drinks.[5]

Wurtman had been hired as a consultant to G.D. Searle and Co., NutraSweet's manufacturer. But while working with Searle, Wurtman found and reported on the seizure cases. These people had never had seizures before. There was no reason why they should have had seizures, except for the effect Wurtman suspected NutraSweet had on their brain cells. The company did not listen to Wurtman's concerns. He came to believe that Searle was not particularly interested in what he had to say.

Wurtman believed the company was not honestly dealing with the safety issue. "I still trust them as far as I can throw your building," he wrote to Sanford A. Miller, of the Food and Drug Administration. As the case reports of seizures accumulated, Wurtman became more and more concerned about the connection between NutraSweet and seizures.

"I thought this was more than a chance coincidence," Wurtman said, "because there are good reasons why aspartame might be expected to make people more likely to have seizures. It contains phenylalanine. When you consume aspartame, something happens to your blood and your brain that never previously happened in man's evolutionary history. It was only after somebody invented a food like aspartame that it was possible to do the experiment asking, when you raise phenylalanine in the brain, what happens? It's an experiment that I think I would rather not have seen done. Because, of all the amino acids, phenylalanine is the one for which there is the best evidence of neurotoxicity."

Phenylalanine can damage brain cells. High levels of phenylalanine develop in children with a disease called phenylketonuria, or PKU. Profound brain damage is often the result. When we consume aspartame, we are essentially drinking phenylalanine. How much NutraSweet can we consume and still be sure that the phenylalanine levels in the brain are safe? No one knows. Wurtman advises pregnant women and small children to stay off aspartame completely. Phenylalanine affects brain cells directly and interferes with substances in the brain which are responsible for preventing seizures.

"We now have over 200 cases of previously healthy young adults who had a full grand mal seizure associated with consuming, over a period of time, large amounts of aspartame," Wurtman said. "Many of these people first have headaches, deja vu, or other symptoms before seizures begin."

Canadian researchers studied children who had had seizures previously, unrelated to aspartame. They found that the chemical made their brain wave patterns even more abnormal, suggesting that it might make existing seizures worse.[6]

At Children's Hospital in Washington, D.C., Dr. C. Keith Conners conducted sophisticated studies on how various nutrients affect children. Conners has found that NutraSweet can cause a variety of physical complaints: headaches, nausea, lethargy, diarrhea, and stomach aches. But it can also produce behavioral effects. One four-year-old had a particularly serious reaction.

> *"We now have over 200 cases of previously healthy young adults who had a full grand mal seizure associated with consuming, over a period of time, large amounts of aspartame."*
>
> *Dr. Richard Wurtman*

"The boy exhibited a profound hyperactivity that came on very suddenly. He became overactive for 36 to 48 hours and didn't sleep, hardly ate, became agitated and quite wild, and had to be restrained. He ran full-tilt into the wall, repeatedly knocking himself down. He became so agitated. This happened on several occasions. Even after he was restricted from all aspartame-containing foods, when he inadvertently received some, the episodes were repeated." If he had Kool-Aid sweetened with sugar there was no problem. But Kool-Aid with NutraSweet caused the bizarre symptoms to recur.

The problems don't end there. "It's turning out that if you open a can of diet soda," Dr. Wurtman said, "you find in that can a lot more than just the aspartame you put in. The chemical is very unstable. By the time you open the can, five to ten percent of it has rearranged to an entirely different chemical called beta-aspartame. Does it enter the brain? I don't know. No one's ever studied it. Now there are seven compounds that people are aware of that are present in the can of soda to which aspartame had been added."

> *"It turning out that if you open a can of diet soda, you find a lot more than just the aspartame you put in. Five to ten percent of it has rearranged to an entirely different chemical.*
>
> **Dr. Richard Wurtman**

Unfortunately, the marketing of aspartame has been full speed ahead, and industry has had little interest in the consequences. "They're just very flagrantly dishonest," Wurtman said. "They lead the listener to believe that phenylalanine is phenylalanine, whether you get it in protein or you get it in aspartame, and that simply isn't true."

Many other researchers have begun to look at the effects of aspartame, and have found mixed results. Many have concluded that it is safe.[7] On the other hand, it is now apparent that supplementing individual amino acids can be dangerous. In the body, aspartame breaks down chemically to its two amino acids, plus a bit of methanol. It is safe to say that no one needs any of these as dietary supplements.

How You Eat Affects How You Sleep

A good night's sleep cures a myriad of ills. In dreams we turn over the troubles of the previous day and put them aside. Our muscles rest, and our body chemistry completes its many nocturnal tasks. When we sleep well, we are ready to take on the next day. When sleep is disrupted, though, we are irritable and easily fatigued. Physical and emotional pains hurt more.

Many people report that dietary habits affect their sleep. For example, large meals late in the evening sometimes interfere with sleep. A lighter dinner earlier in the evening may help. In addition, we can manipulate the brain's chemistry to promote a good night's sleep. *Serotonin* is a natural chemical in the brain. Among many other functions, serotonin acts as a hypnotic. When serotonin is more plentiful, we feel sleepy. The concentration of serotonin in the brain depends on the balance of proteins and carbohydrates in the foods we eat.

Pure carbohydrate meals increase serotonin. Carbohydrates are sugars or combinations of sugars. A piece of cake or pie or a glass of juice before bed increases the amount of serotonin in the brain and helps us sleep. The sandman would be more effective if he would leave his sand at home and distribute jelly donuts instead.

But this effect is blocked by protein. If there is much protein in the foods we have eaten, serotonin levels will not rise, and the sedative effect will not occur. So to feel sleepy, have a high-carbohydrate snack, such as fruit juice or cake. To avoid drowsiness after meals, have a mixture of carbohydrate and protein.

In the morning, we want to feel alert. So we will block the carbohydrate effect with a small amount of protein. A mixture of protein and carbohydrate has none of the serotonin-enhancing effect of pure carbohydrate. Very little protein is needed to block the carbohydrate effect. If protein makes up about ten percent of the meal, the effect is blocked.[8] Happily, most foods contain both protein and carbohydrate. Oatmeal, for example, contains both, as do other breakfast cereals and whole wheat toast. These foods contain enough protein to block the serotonin effect.

The usual American breakfast has a large amount of protein in eggs, bacon, and sausage, but these foods have an enormous content of fat and cholesterol. In Mexico and parts of England, a breakfast may consist of beans on toast. While it sounds odd to Americans, this breakfast is a way of combining protein (far more than is needed to block the carbohydrate effect) with carbohydrate, while eliminating the unwanted fat and cholesterol.

How Carbohydrate Works

The brain makes many of the chemicals it needs from proeins. A protein molecule is like a string of beads. When we digest proteins, the "beads" come off, each bead being an amino acid molecule. It is these amino acids that are used to build what the body needs.

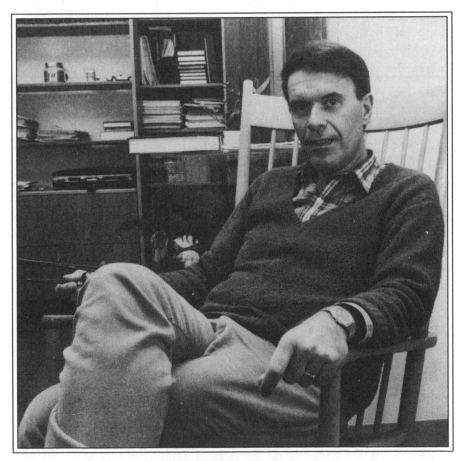

Dr. Richard Wurtman

The brain makes serotonin from a particular amino acid called tryptophan. The more tryptophan that passes from the blood stream into the brain, the more serotonin it makes. But the brain does not automatically get as much tryptophan as it can use. Only so many amino acid molecules can pass from the blood stream into the brain at a time. Tryptophan is competing with the other amino acids to get into the brain.

Here is where carbohydrate works. Carbohydrate stimulates the release of insulin, which ushers many of the competing amino acids out of the blood stream. (Insulin also does the same to sugar.) Tryptophan is left behind because it is attached to a carrier molecule which prevents it from leaving the blood. Now it has less competition for getting into the brain, where it can produce serotonin.

It is a complicated path, but it works: carbohydrate increases insulin, which increases the amount of tryptophan that gets to the brain, which increases serotonin, which makes us fall asleep. Studies have shown that the same regimen can raise the pain threshold, so that hurts hurt a little less. [9,10]

Dr. Wurtman had originally thought that protein would increase tryptophan levels in the brain. After all, protein contains tryptophan as one of its amino acid building blocks. But he found that protein did not increase the amount of tryptophan getting to the brain. Sometimes, in fact, it actually reduced it. "It took us a while before we acknowledged it," Wurtman said, "because the experiments didn't work the way we expected them to. And the reason is this: Protein contains some tryptophan. But it contains a much larger amount of the other amino acids that compete with tryptophan." There is just too much competition. There are no foods that supply tryptophan without an overly generous supply of its competitors.

"There was an article in the *New York Times* saying that if you want to feel sleepy, eat tryptophan, and the way to do that is by having turkey," Wurtman said. "I sent them a letter and they published a correction. There is no protein source that will raise brain tryptophan. All natural proteins contain so little tryptophan compared with the other amino acids that they have either no effect or they lower brain tryptophan.

"You have to eat carbohydrate. You can use carbohydrate like a drug, up to a point. You can decide that for a few hours you would like to increase your brain serotonin, because you want to go to sleep, or because you feel jittery or what have you. I know a number of people who do quite well having a piece of cake and some orange juice at bedtime. It has a very nice effect."

Food and Your Mood

Depression is a condition of the mind and the body, causing sleeplessness, apathy, loss of energy, inability to make decisions, and suicidal thoughts. Interest in food changes as well. A loss of appetite often occurs, although, for some, appetite increases.

Chemical neurotransmitters—the messengers by which brain cells communicate with each other—are the pathways through which experiences lead to depression or other feelings. It is also through these neurotransmitter chemicals that antidepressant medications exert their effect. Too little of a certain neurotransmitter, and we feel like a sinking ship. Too much, and we feel revved up. Two neurotransmitter chemicals are particularly important in depression: serotonin, which we have seen is also a regulator of sleep, and norepinephrine, a close relative of adrenaline. Antidepressant medications increase the levels of these natural brain chemicals. Nutrients can, to an extent, do the same thing.

Some people have what may be a natural deficiency of serotonin. They are often depressed, particularly in the winter months when there is less daylight. This annual cycle of depression is termed Seasonal Affective Disorder (SAD). Many people with SAD crave carbohydrates, perhaps as a natural way to increase serotonin in the brain. The carbohydrates need not be sweet. Starchy carbohydrates are craved as well and raise serotonin just as effectively.

A research study at the Massachusetts Institute of Technology compared two groups of overweight people: "carbohydrate cravers" and those who do not have this tendency. After a meal of pure carbohydrates, those who were not carbohydrate cravers often felt worse. It made them sleepy or irritable. But the carbohydrate cravers had a very different reaction to the pure carbohydrate meals.

"It did not make them sleepy or grumpy," Wurtman said. "It actually improved their mood significantly. It's tempting to speculate that carbohydrate cravers, perhaps, don't have enough serotonin for whatever reason."

The carbohydrate-seeking behavior appears to be a way to restore serotonin balance. So carbohydrate cravers feel better after a carbohydrate meal. Others, however, feel worse, unless the carbohydrate is mixed with proteins.

We've seen how serotonin is affected by the balance of carbohydrate and protein in our diet. Researchers are also studying ways to increase norepinephrine with food. Norepinephrine is made from another common amino acid, called tyrosine. Tyrosine is found in many proteins, but eating these proteins will not have much of an effect on the amount that gets to the brain, because, again, competition with other amino acids keeps large amounts of any one from gaining access to the brain. High-carbohydrate diets will raise norepinephrine production somewhat, as we saw in Chapter 4.

Some researchers have used pure tyrosine as an experimental antidepressant. Used alone, it is not very potent. It does not work at all in brain cells which are relatively inactive. Only when brain cells are actively communicating with each other do they use tyrosine to make more norepinephrine. Some research indicates that tyrosine works best when given along with tryptophan. This combination mimics the effect of antidepressant medications, most of which increase both norepinephrine and serotonin in the brain.

By a related mechanism, tyrosine may be helpful in Parkinson's disease, a syndrome in which normal movements are disrupted by tremor and muscular rigidity. A deficiency of the neurotransmitter dopamine plays an important role in this disease. Dopamine is also made from tyrosine. Research has shown some benefits from tyrosine for some patients with Parkinson's disease. It does not appear to be a substitute for more established treatments, but may have an adjunctive role.

Many people with Parkinson's disease also benefit from a dietary plan in which virtually no protein is eaten until evening. Researchers at Georgetown University in Washington, D.C., have shown that by consuming fruits and other low-protein foods during the day and reserving higher-protein foods for the evening, medications had an improved effect.

For now, all we have are hints as to what tyrosine can do. How much we can use it to manipulate brain chemistry is not yet clear. Again, do not use tyrosine or any other concentrated amino acid without a physician's supervision.

Riding the Sugar Roller Coaster

Sugar is a simple carbohydrate. Some people have a very negative reaction to sugar, as the case below illustrates:

> *A hard-working businesswoman was concerned about moody episodes. She was always productive at her job and was an active, outgoing person. But every now and then she had days when she felt entirely out of sorts. She was tired, and tired of people. She felt overly irritated with subordinates and annoyed at her friends. These episodes did not seem to relate to any particular event. They did not relate to how much sleep she had had, or with her menstrual cycle, or anything else she could think of. But they seemed to last for the whole day, or even a couple of days.*
>
> *She wondered if her diet was the culprit. She had a habit of stopping at a coffee shop on the way to work for some sugared donuts and had sugary sweets occasionally at other times. She began to suspect that the irritability and fatigue were related to the sugar. She stopped eating refined sugars altogether for about a month and found that she never had these episodes. She then challenged herself with sugar again and felt characteristically irritable. She continued to stay away from sugar and has felt fine.*

Why was she irritable after having carbohydrates, such as sugar? Possibly because the carbohydrate was driving up her serotonin levels. For many people, especially at night, that is fine. But many of us feel irritable and tired after the serotonin-raising effect of pure-carbohydrate foods. The effect can be blocked by choosing a mix of foods—meals that contain both protein and carbohydrate. From a practical standpoint, that means avoiding sugary foods. Instead, emphasize whole foods which contain a natural balance of nutrients: grains, legumes, and vegetables.

For children, sugar does more than cause cavities. It clearly affects the way the brain works. Sometimes sugar makes children inattentive and diminishes their ability to think and react. Under certain circumstances, however, sugar actually helps brain function. The key is in what else the child has eaten.

At Children's Hospital in Washington D. C., Conners tested the effects of sugar on children. If children had had a mainly carbohydrate breakfast, such as plain white toast, a sugar snack later in the day would impair their attention span and slow their reaction time. But if the breakfast contained more protein, sugar actually improved mental functioning. The carbohydrate breakfast probably led to an increase in serotonin levels in the brain. Sugar aggravated this effect. But adding protein to the breakfast could block the effect.

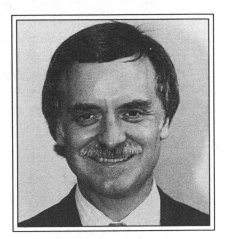

The amount of sugar Conners used in the study was considerable—about the amount combined in a large piece of cherry pie and a chocolate candy bar. This is a sizable

Dr. C. Keith Conners

quantity, but not out of the range of many children's eating habits.

Conners showed that the effects of sugar could even be seen in brain waves measured on the electroencephalogram (EEG). "In one of the tests we had electrodes attached to the scalp so we could measure the brain response," he said. "We know that the brain is normally asymmetrical and that the two hemispheres of the brain function quite differently. Verbal functions, on the whole, are on one side of the brain and spatial functions are on the other side. In this case, the asymmetry that is normally there was abolished by the carbohydrate. It was as though one side of the brain had been compromised by this temporary load.

"Sugar has its largest effect within an hour," Conners said, "but the effects continue throughout the morning. A child whose reaction was slowed gets even slower during the later part of the day, even though the blood sugar has returned to normal." But the effect was totally offset by having protein at breakfast. With protein and sugar together, the children Conners studied did very well.

What about fruit sugars, that is, the fructose in fruit and in honey? Conners found fructose no better than table sugar. "We compared fructose with sucrose (table sugar) and didn't really see any notable behavioral differences," Conners said. "In the lay literature, fructose is seen to be the 'good sugar,' particularly in the form of honey, and sucrose is the 'bad sugar.' In fact, you're probably doing more harm to yourself by eating honey from all the junk which is cooked in with it than you are by eating pure table sugar."

Children need breakfasts which combine carbohydrate and protein. Oatmeal or wheat cereals, for example, naturally combine both protein and carbohydrate.

Hyperactivity and the Feingold Diet

Hyperactive children are often restless and fidgety. They may run and climb at a pace that would exhaust other children. They may do poorly in school, which is often wrongly attributed to misbehavior.

The current diagnostic term for this syndrome is Attention Deficit Disorder, because one of the most common findings is an inability to focus attention for more than a brief period. Learning disabilities are also common in these children. Subtle abnormalities of the brain are probably responsible for the hyperactivity and the learning troubles these children experience.

In the 1970s, Dr. Ben Feingold popularized a dietary treatment for hyperactivity. Feingold, a pediatric allergist, noticed that the increasing incidence of hyperactivity in America paralleled the increasing use of artificial flavors and colors in foods. He hypothesized that hyperactivity was caused by a sensitivity to these additives and devised a diet that eliminated them. In addition, because some people who are allergic to food dyes are also sensitive to aspirin and related compounds, called salicylates, he also eliminated salicylate-containing foods, such as tomatoes, cucumbers, and fruits. With his diet, Feingold found dramatic improvements in the behavior of hyperactive children. As many as two-thirds of hyperactive children improved.

Feingold published his findings in *Why Your Child is Hyperactive* (Random House, 1985). As his interest in hyperactivity developed, one of the researchers whose works he read was Keith Conners. In turn, Conners tested Feingold's hypothesis.

At first, it appeared that Feingold was right. Conners confirmed that about two-thirds of children seemed to improve on the diet. But Conners became concerned that it was not the diet that was helping, but rather the parents' expectation that the children should improve. So he did another study, using hidden food additives. He gave children two kinds of cookies. Some contained food dye. Others were placebo cookies with no food dye.

"The mother of the very first patient called up the next day after receiving the cookie and said, 'I don't know what you put in that cookie, but whatever it is, I'm taking the kid out of the study, because he has gone berserk. He took a hammer and went next door and beat up the neighbor's motorcycle, he cut up our couch and just went wild. So those food dyes you put in that cookie are driving him crazy, and I'm taking him out of the study.' Well, as luck would have it, that child received placebo cookies the first day. He was responding to his own expectations of what ought to be happening when he eats a bad thing."

So is the Feingold diet just a placebo? "If you just put everybody on the diet, absolutely two-thirds of them get remarkably better," Conners said. "As soon as you do it in a double-blind fashion, those effects disappear. So it really means that if a person believes in the treatment, they will get better. It's largely a placebo effect. Feingold was misled by these rather dramatic changes into thinking they were real because he didn't believe that placebos could be that effective.

Placebos are very powerful. When they're not controlled, they mislead even the best scientific observers. Dr. Feingold was a true humanist and a very genuine and committed man, but he essentially dropped his scientific guard at the wrong time."

That does not mean that the Feingold diet is totally ineffective. There does seem to be a small group of children who do, in fact, respond well to the diet. "In almost all the studies there have been one or two kids where there seems to be a pretty regular effect," Conners said. "We found when we started using more sensitive measures that there were a few such kids, usually younger kids."

Conners urges, though, that medical problems and the Feingold diet not be used as reasons to avoid looking at problems in the family that may be contributing to a child's difficulties. "Diets may be used as an argument against changing your own behavior and against examining family process problems that are more subtle and perhaps important." Foods are a part of the puzzle of hyperactivity, taking their place along with other pieces that are also important.

Metals and Brain Function

Lead causes brain damage. In children, even subtle brain damage from lead can cause hyperactivity, learning disabilities, or mental retardation. There may be no symptoms to indicate that lead poisoning was the cause, and unless a pediatrician checks for lead in the blood (a simple test), lead poisoning can continue undetected indefinitely. Lead can also damage the kidneys and cause abdominal and muscular symptoms.

Where does lead come from? Lead can enter the body insidiously in foods, in drinking water, and even in the air we breathe. A nursing mother with high lead levels will secrete lead in her milk.

"Kids are actually exposed to lead quite a bit," Dr. Conners said. "There's lead in the ground; there's lead in the air; there's lead in pipes; there's lead in the solders that are used to repair pipes." In fact, the word plumbing comes from the Latin word *plumbum* which means lead, the original metal from which pipes were made. Lead pipes and solder joints are still found in homes. Leaded paints are still on the walls of many old homes. High lead levels have been detected in as many as twenty percent of children, particularly in poor neighborhoods.

Dietary deficiencies also play a role, as Conners explains. "A poor mother is more likely to be a working mother. She doesn't have the luxury of breast-feeding until the child is eight or nine months or a year of age. Instead, from a very early age the child finds himself eating out of a bottle while the mother is going to work. The child then doesn't get the nutrients which are in breast milk. He is more likely to develop iron deficiency." A lack of iron can lead to more than anemia. Iron, like other minerals, helps prevent lead from entering the gut or the brain. It competes against lead. Without iron, lead can enter the brain more easily. A healthy diet, with an adequate amount of iron, helps keep lead out of the brain.

> *"Kids are actually exposed to lead quite a bit. There's lead in the ground; there's lead in the air; there's lead in pipes; there's lead in the solders that are used to repair pipes."*
>
> **Dr. C. Keith Conners**

But even in children who are well-nourished, foods may play a role in protecting the brain from lead. A recent study showed a surprising connection between intelligence and the amount of whole wheat bread in the diet. Children who ate more whole wheat bread were found to have higher scores on IQ tests. It turned out that they were less likely to have lead poisoning than children who ate white bread. Why? "Zinc, which is in the kernel of the wheat bread, is removed from the white," Conners said. "A preference for white bread lowered zinc levels, which made lead exposure more toxic and therefore lowered the IQ." In addition, the fiber in whole wheat bread probably helps remove lead from the digestive tract, so less is absorbed.

"When we've looked at the diets of children who come to our impatient psychiatric service for severe behavioral problems," Conners said, "they have tremendously poor diets. They eat everything under the sun, including garbage and soil and wallpaper and paint and very little of what they're supposed to be eating. In some, we may see a kind of uninhibited, impulsive availability of foods that taste good. That tends to predispose them to soft drinks, to quick-energy foods, to sweet foods. These things are not bad in themselves; it's the excess and the fact that they crowd out the other foods that one needs."

In the not too distant past there was another source of lead: automobile exhaust. A study in Canada gave compelling evidence that lead from auto exhaust can cause hyperactivity. "They drew a map of the prevalence of hyperactivity using one of these contour maps that is used to visualize mountain ranges, but instead of mountain ranges the elevations represented numbers of hyperactive children," Conners said. "They found a 'mountain range' of hyperactivity running right down the center of Ottawa along the Queen's Highway. The lead levels in the soil for 200 yards on either side of the highway were significantly raised. There are also studies in New York of children who were exposed to lead, and their hyperactivity was reduced once the lead was lowered in the blood."

> *"When we've looked at the diets of children who come to our inpatient psychiatric service for severe behavioral problems, they have tremendously poor diets."*
>
> **Dr. C. Keith Conners**

Children who grew up near major highways were at risk for lead poisoning and brain damage. Restrictions on leaded gasoline have diminished this problem. Drinking water should be tested for lead. In addition, foods may play an important role. Breast-feeding for infants and high-fiber foods such as whole wheat bread may help prevent lead from entering the brain.

Another element, boron, may improve brain function. Apples, pears, grapes, and leafy vegetables contain generous amounts of boron, which has been shown to improve alertness by psychologist James C. Penland and his colleagues at the Agricultural Research Service in Grand Forks, North Dakota. Meats and dairy products contain virtually no boron.

Alzheimer's Disease

An executive who retired about five years ago came to see his doctor at his wife's request. He seemed to be forgetful, she said, and the gaps in his memory were becoming gradually more common. He recognized this, but attributed it to "the dull life of retirement." He tried to cover over his lapses by joking about them or changing the subject. He had never been good with names, but found that now he often forgot names he was sure he knew. He began to have trouble with simple arithmetic. Counting change became an impossible task. Eventually, he found that when he got to the end of a newspaper article, he had forgotten the beginning.

His wife was right to have him see his doctor. Memory problems can be due to treatable conditions, such as depression, heart disease, medications, or other problems. Unfortunately, he was not so lucky. No treatable cause of his illness could be found. His doctor made a tentative diagnosis of Alzheimer's disease. Very gradually he lost more and more of his capacity to care for himself. He eventually moved to a nursing home where he died a few years later.

One and one-half to two million Americans have Alzheimer's disease. Its main characteristic is dementia, that is, the loss of intellectual capacities. For some, the illness occurs early, between about 40 and 60 years of age. For others, the disease occurs only late in life.

The search for causes has turned up some interesting leads. People with Alzheimer's disease have been found to have aluminum in their brains. Autopsies showed that aluminum concentrates in the parts of the brain most affected by the disease. Is aluminum the cause? No one knows. Perhaps aluminum has nothing to do with causing the disease and was simply drawn to the damaged parts of the brain. But it may well be that aluminum actually does the damage.

"Unfortunately, we still don't know the answer," Wurtman said. "We do have more reason to worry now, I think. In the last few years very compelling data have been adduced showing a clear relationship between aluminum silicate and the two cardinal lesions of Alzheimer's disease, namely the plaques and tangles in the brain." Plaques and neurofibrillary tangles are microscopic abnormalities found in the brains of patients with Alzheimer's disease.

"If you analyze brain samples from people who have died of Alzheimer's disease, there's a very tight association between aluminum and the neurofibrillary tangles. A group of investigators recently found the same thing with plaques. So the question is, is it that the sick cell somehow attracts and binds aluminum? Or is aluminum somehow involved in causing the sickness? And here I don't think one knows the answer."

> *"In the last few years very compelling data have been adduced showing a clear relationship between aluminum silicate and the two cardinal lesions of Alzheimer's disease."*
>
> **Dr. Richard Wurtman**

Until we know more we should be careful about aluminum. The main sources of aluminum are certain antacids, aluminum cans and cookware, and some processed cheeses. It is certainly easy to live without each of these. There is also a small amount of aluminum in common table salt and other packaged foods.

There is also evidence that people with Alzheimer's disease have too little of a neurotransmitter chemical, *acetylcholine*, in the brain. Research studies have looked at ways of stimulating acetylcholine production through diet. These have relied on giving nutrients called *choline* and *phosphatidylcholine* (also called *lecithin*), which the brain turns into acetylcholine. Some investigators have suggested that if lecithin is given long enough, it may slow or stop the progression of the disease for some patients, particularly older patients.

These supplements may work by stopping the destruction of brain cells. Brain cells that are hungry for acetylcholine may actually take choline from their own cell membranes in order to make it, a process referred to as "autocannibalism." "It may be that autocannibalism is part of the process of Alzheimer's disease," Wurtman said. "When you give people supplemental choline, then they stop breaking down their own membranes. Some might get a little bit better too, either because you've saved some sick membranes or because you have increased acetylcholine release from them."

Where do we find choline in the diet? "You find very little free choline," Wurtman said, "except in a few vegetables like cauliflower, which is rich in choline. But most of the choline you find in the diet is in the form of phosphatidylcholine or lecithin, which is present in eggs and glandular meats, like liver. It's present in soybeans. It's used as an emulsifying agent in chocolate."

Eggs and organ meats are very high in cholesterol, and should be avoided. It would certainly be unwise to try to counteract Alzheimer's disease with foods that may promote a stroke or heart attack. Cauliflower is safe on both counts. But purified lecithin is what current research relies on. Researchers on Alzheimer's disease use doses of lecithin that are far higher than those available in foods.

"I hasten to add that one should not run off to the health food store and buy lecithin there," Wurtman said. "Even if it's called pure lecithin, by a quirk in the labeling laws, it will contain perhaps only 20 percent lecithin or less. But now several companies are making purified lecithin in the form of capsules or food-based preparations available to psychiatrists.

"Most people probably consume on the order of maybe 200 to 400 milligrams of choline per day. The doses of lecithin that are used in the study of Alzheimer's disease probably supply two to three grams of choline per day. By taking a large amount of purified lecithin, you're going to have an effect on brain acetylcholine, and ameliorate some conditions which seem to be related to increased acetylcholine."

Stroke

A stroke can be devastating. In a stroke, part of the brain is destroyed.

A 48-year-old stockbroker was in excellent physical condition. He enjoyed competitive tennis and golf. He played with his children and often took the family sailing. But one day, while getting up from his desk, his right leg suddenly went limp. He collapsed and hit the floor hard. He could not get up. He found that his right hand and arm would not function. Try as he might, he could not move even a single finger.

He had had an episode a month earlier in which his right leg became suddenly weak, but it passed very quickly. He had thought nothing about it at the time. Now, his limbs seemed totally lifeless.

He tried to call out, but found he could not speak. He could make moaning sounds, but could not form words. He could not even think of which words to say. He felt completely helpless. He wondered if he were dreaming and would wake up fully restored.

Unfortunately, he was not dreaming. He had had a typical stroke. This sort of event happens to a half a million Americans each year. Most stroke victims are older than this young man. But strokes can hit people in their thirties or even younger.

What destroyed his ability to function was very simple. Atherosclerotic plaques—patches of cholesterol, fat, and cells—had gradually developed in the arteries leading to his brain. The passageway for blood became narrower and narrower. One day, an artery on the left side of his brain closed off completely, perhaps by a blood clot lodged in the narrow passageway. On the left side of the brain is the control center for the right arm and leg. Near it is the center for speech. In an instant, these areas were choked off.

In the next several weeks, he slowly recovered his speech. But his arm and leg remained weak for the rest of his life. Although he had been in top physical condition, the progress of atherosclerosis had been continuing unseen in his arteries.

Dementia that resembles Alzheimer's disease may sometimes be due to strokes. Many small, undetectable strokes can occur over months or years, each one killing a small part of the brain. Mental functions deteriorate in a step-wise fashion as parts of the brain are sequentially killed off. The final result is dementia, a major deterioration in mental function.

In people who have had a loss of mental abilities, it may be difficult to tell whether the cause is Alzheimer's disease or the progression of many small strokes. A computerized tomography (CT) scan can demonstrate the hole in the brain caused by a large stroke, but small strokes will often not be visible.

Strokes are often preventable. They occur when a plaque or blood clot lodges in an artery of the brain, or when plaques expand and close off the artery, or when an artery bursts. Sometimes congenitally malformed blood vessels will lead to a stroke.

Prevention follows the same process as the prevention of heart disease: stay away from foods rich in fat and cholesterol, avoid tobacco, and keep blood pressure under control. Fats and cholesterol are principally in meats and dairy products. A shift from these foods to foods from plant sources—beans, grains, vegetables, and fruits—is important.

The Mind's Eye on the Dinner Plate

Why should nature have allowed the brain to be battered about by something as trivial as our last meal? Why should carbohydrates and proteins be able to change neurotransmitter levels in the brain? It appears that this is the brain's way of monitoring our dietary intake. The brain tells us when to start or stop eating and what kinds of foods to select, often with great specificity. Neurotransmitters play a part in this regulatory process and change depending on what we are eating.

"If you were to count up all the foods you eat per week," Wurtman said, "and determine what percentage of the calories come from protein or carbohydrate, you'd find remarkable stability. And you are totally unaware of that. Well, your brain isn't. You think you are eating because the food smells good or because it's time to eat. To some extent you are. But in reality, your brain is choosing nutrients.

"I think that this mechanism was chosen by evolution in order, for instance, to keep the bear from only eating honey. Certain things taste very good, and that's dangerous. If the bear just ate honey, he wouldn't be a healthy bear."

Unfortunately, although our brain carefully balances our selections of carbohydrate and protein, it does not protect us from eating things that are unhealthy. The biggest problem seems to be the amount of fat we consume. Nearly half our calories each day come from fat. We choose fatty hamburgers, fried chicken, french fries, and other greasy foods. These selections, never vetoed by the brain, lead to heart disease, cancer, an epidemic of obesity, and numerous other problems. Although people have searched for connections between fatty foods and the brain from many years (Sir Andrew in Shakespear's *Twelfth Night*

> *"You think you are eating because the food smells good, or because it's time to eat. But in reality, your brain is choosing nutrients. I think that this mechanism was chosen by evolution in order to keep the bear from only eating honey."*
>
> **Dr. Richard Wurtman**

said, "I am a great eater of beef and I believe it does harm to my wit."), these relationships are not yet elucidated. There does not seem to be a neurochemical that is automatically affected by fat in the diet. So, unfortunately, fat comes along for the ride. If our brain is seeking out carbohydrate and chooses ice cream, then a lot of fat will be part of the meal. If on the other hand, it chooses rice as the source of carbohydrate, very little fat will be consumed. "Through our evolution this was not much of a problem," Wurtman said, "because fat was always very expensive. People did not have the capacity, unless they killed a walrus or something, of having enormous amounts of fat. But now fat is so cheap and available that we find large amounts of it present with the carbohydrates and proteins that we eat. And I really think that's the problem."

Fat is often craved in its many forms. At a previous time in our evolution, this made sense. Fat is a calorie-dense food. A gram of fat has more than twice the calories (nine) of a gram of carbohydrate or protein (four). By taking advantage of fatty foods on those rare occasions when they were available, our ancestors found a rich source of calories. But now that is the last thing we need. At the end of this book we'll see how it is possible to turn down our fat-seeking behavior. By consistently eating fewer fatty foods, the amount of fat desired (or tolerated) can be diminished.

Remembering Our Dietary Past

Prior to a century or two ago, the production of foods was a very different process than it is today. Flours were largely unrefined. Refined sugars were less available. Aluminum-containing antacids were not on our shelves. NutraSweet was not something we thought we needed.

Dietary traditions have often been ritualized in cultural practices. In the Jain culture in India, for example, food is not consumed after dark. While this is for several reasons, it is likely to minimize the disruption of sleep that may occur after a large meal.

Conners said, "In most religions, at what I would call their highest level, the level of the inner circle of practitioners, the same proscriptions about diet have obtained. Whether you're Moslem, Jewish, Buddhist, or Mormon, they all preach moderation and using food in a very skillful way to augment your main life goal. They also tend, on the whole, to dislike killing and to have proscriptions against animal food."

There is some value to recalling the past. For most of our history, animal foods were a smaller part of the diet. Strokes and heart disease were correspondingly less common. Without refining, foods contained a helpful balance of nutrients. The effect on amino acid levels, and therefore on neurotransmitters, was likely to have been more balanced. Our fragile brain cells were less often assaulted by unfamiliar chemicals and better protected when assaults occurred.

Chapter 8

The Evolution of the Human Diet

The clear waters of Lake Tanganyika reach to the shores of Gombe, a strip of rugged, beautiful country in the Kigoma region of Tanzania. It was here in Gombe that Jane Goodall came in July, 1960, to study chimpanzees at the suggestion of paleoanthropologist Louis Leakey. Her studies of chimpanzees and what they eat tell us much about the natural diet of the human animal. There is also human evidence of our dietary development, as we will learn from Leakey's famous son, Richard. But first, let's take a brief look at our primate relatives and the earlier stages of our own dietary evolution.

For some time after Dr. Goodall's arrival, the chimpanzees cautiously avoided her approach. She had to observe at a distance through binoculars. But gradually the chimpanzees discovered there was nothing to fear and accepted the human tag-along. Eventually she took on field assistants and students who helped with observations and reporting in what was to become the longest continuous field study of any living creature. In the process, she has come to know the chimpanzees as individuals. Each has a unique life story Goodall has been able to observe. Chimps have been born. Others have died. Affection and playfulness, power struggles, and keen awareness of social structure are ingrained in chimpanzee life.

Fruits, Seeds, and Medicinal Plants

Millions of years ago, our history was merged with that of chimpanzees. Our common ancestors lived in Africa, eating what the African climate provided. What did our primate ancestors eat? Was it Spam and roast beef sandwiches? Frozen yogurt? Kidney pie? If we can judge from the chimpanzees, it was mostly fruit.

Fruits typically make up more than half of the chimps' diet. Goodall's notes contain vivid descriptions, such as Passion, the careless chimp who did not bother to wipe off the mess of sticky juice from the strychnos fruits she had been eating, while seated next to her, her three-year-old son, Pax, meticulously wiped his chin clean with blades of grass.

"The chimps spend a great deal of time eating the fruit that is in season," Goodall said. "Probably the most significant is the fruit of the oil nut palm, because the trees have their own individual cycles. The fruit clusters ripen one after the other throughout the year, so the chimps can get palm nuts in virtually any month."

Just as human civilizations develop their culturally favorite foods, chimps do the same. These traditions are passed

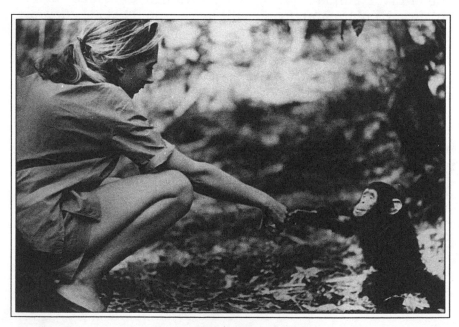

Dr. Jane Goodall and friend

from parent to child in each succeeding generation.

"The oil nut palm is the most dramatic example," Goodall said. "The Gombe chimps eat the fruit; they eat the pith; they eat the dried male flower cluster—at least they chew and spit out the fiber; and they also eat the dead wood from the trunk. At Mahale, by contrast, chimps don't eat any part of this palm. In the Tai Forest of the Ivory Coast the chimps have not been seen eating the palm nuts. They do, however, commonly eat the pith. In Liberia, they crack open the hard kernels using stone hammers and eat the nuts inside; these are not eaten at Gombe or at Tai.

"There are differences in methods of feeding as well. The chimps at Gombe eat the strychnos fruit by cracking it open against a stone, and the Mahale chimps break open the fruit with their teeth. So there are very clear cultural differences between different populations.

"I suspect that new cultural traditions of this sort are mostly started by infants," Goodall said, "because infants are the ones who are always exploring, testing, trying. Sometimes an adult will actually prevent an infant from feeding on a fruit that is not a part of the adult diet, even though we know it not to be poisonous. When I offered new foods to infants, they were usually interested, but sometimes others prevented them from actually eating them. An elder sister flicked biscuit crumbs away from her infant brother, a mother seized a piece of papaya from her child, sniffed it, then hurled it away, and so on."

After fruits, leaves are the next largest part of the diet, comprising 10 to 40 percent of the chimpanzee menu, followed by seeds and blossoms. The chimps have even found a medicinal leaf, the aspilia leaf. "There is evidently an antibiotic in these leaves,"Goodall said. "Instead of chewing them, the chimp sort of rubs them against the roof of his mouth with his tongue, then swallows them whole."

The aspilia leaves have been shown to contain a natural chemical that helps prevent infections. Many human cultures have also made use of the aspilia leaves in medicines. The chimps may have made similar discoveries in wood and bark. They chew the fibers to extract the juices. Is it simply recreation, or is there some natural kind of medicine in the plant fibers? Few of the extracts have been analyzed, and, unlike humans, chimpanzees have no distinction between foods and medicines. "Perhaps some of the foods the chimps eat would be quite beneficial to humans," Goodall said, "from a nutritional as well as medical point of view."

On their diet of fruits and vegetation, the chimps remain amazingly healthy, free of most of the diseases that plague humans.

Meat-Eating

Chimpanzees, like other primates, eat a mainly vegetarian diet. Dairy products, beef, and poultry are never eaten by our evolutionary cousins. From time to time, however, they eat insects, and even kill small mammals, typically infant colobus monkeys. Although only a tiny percentage of the chimpanzees diet (four percent or less, varying widely from month to month) consists of meat, Goodall's work has given surprising glimpses of hunting behavior of chimpanzees.

"In some months, an individual may eat meat six times or more, during others rather less, during some, not at all," Goodall said. "The most frequently eaten prey animal at Gombe is the red colobus monkey. The chimps usually capture the young. But the total amount of meat consumed by a chimpanzee during a given year will represent only a very small percentage of the overall diet."

> *"The total amount of meat consumed by a chimpanzee during a given year will represent only a very small percentage of the overall diet."*
>
> **Dr. Jane Goodall**

Hunting is usually a group effort. "When the chimps encounter a colobus troop they often sit quietly and gaze up into the treetops," Goodall said. "They are probably noticing how many young ones there are, the whereabouts of the adult males, and so on. They may look at each other, hair bristling, give grins of excitement, make little squeaks or grunts, and reach out to touch one another. Often a number of different chimps start to chase different monkeys at the same time. This causes confusion in the monkey troop. It is then less easy for the adult male monkeys to join forces to intimidate and harass the hunters. A mother will be seized, and her infant snatched away. Colobus monkeys often fall during a hunt. Those chimps waiting on the ground are quick to seize these unfortunate individuals.

"An infant is most often killed as its captor bites into its head. Then death is very quick. But the chimps usually have difficulty in killing adult monkeys or any large prey. Sometimes such victims are dispatched efficiently with a neck bite, but usually by disemboweling which is often slow. Some prey is incapacitated, then killed by eating. It is gruesome to watch."

Females tend to hunt less than do males. One female, however, actually engaged in cannibalism. Passion, at times assisted by her daughter, Pom, attacked other female chimps, seizing and eating their newborn infants.

What can this activity of the chimps show us about the natural diet of humans? First of all, meat-eating must have been much less common in our past than it is today. It is a great deal of trouble for chimpanzees to eat meat, and so it becomes rather rare. If anything, early humans would have eaten meat even less than do the chimpanzees. For while chimps have large canine teeth which can tear apart their prey, humans lost those long ago, long before we invented stone tools that could take their place. Nor do we have even a semblance of the strength and speed of chimps. So, in all probability, we were eating the vegetarian foods available in the forest.

Goodall herself has shifted to a more natural diet. "My diet has changed recently," Goodall said, "just because I've learned too much about factory farming,* and I absolutely refuse to eat meat that comes from a factory-farmed animal or eggs that come from a factory-farmed chicken. I don't mind eating meat so much in Tanzania, where I am in Dar es Salaam, because I know the farmer, and I know his animals are well cared for and humanely slaughtered on the farm. But I find that I actually don't like eating meat anymore."

The Search for Clues to Our Past

There is little doubt that the wide travels which have taken our kind to every part of the globe began in Africa. North

---

Factory farming is the intensive, large-scale process of raising animals for food production that is used in most Western countries today. Animals are confined with little room to move or even turn around, and physical alterations of animals are common to keep them from injuring each other. They are often covered with their own or each other's wastes.

of Gombe, in neighboring Kenya, Richard Leakey searches for clues to the changing anatomy and behavior of our ancestors of millions of years ago. While the evolutionary trail of bones and other remnants which could have told the story of our past was largely devoured in time like the bread crumbs of Hansel and Gretel, a few vital clues remain. In 1967, while flying along the eastern shore of Lake Turkana, Leakey noticed eroded layers of lake deposits which he judged would hold fossils of millions of years ago. He was right. The bones and stone tools that were the remnants of our human ancestors were buried under layer after layer of silt. Erosion has begun to uncover these long-buried clues from the past. The fossil specimens his team has found have been carefully examined. Bones have been analyzed by visual inspection, microscopic examination of surface scratch marks, and other techniques to reveal how humans evolved in the changing environment.

Can we say what made up the diet of early humans? Would our diet have been like that of a chimpanzee, relying on fruits, leaves, seeds, and other vegetation? "The diet of a primate such as a baboon or chimpanzee wouldn't be a bad pattern," Leakey said. "There's an awful lot of food available on the savannah that can be picked with the hands, from fruits, to tubers, to rhizomes, to plants above and below the ground, to insects. There was quite enough food on the African savannah in times of plenty for large primates to be very happy."

Are chimpanzees really a good model for the human diet? How close are we to chimpanzees in an evolutionary sense? "Molecular biologists and geneticists have compared proteins and compared DNA and compared the whole spectrum of biochemical features," Leakey said. "They have established very convincingly that we are closer to the chimpanzee than a horse is to a donkey. We are extraordinarily similar."

But we are also very different. Baboons and chimpanzees have many anatomical differences from hominids, the name used for humans and our human-like predecessors. Chimpanzees have large canine teeth. Early humans, like modern humans, did not. As a result, if we ever caught an animal, tearing through its hide or cutting its flesh would have been an enormous struggle until the invention of stone tools much later. "You can't tear flesh by hand; you can't tear hide by hand," said Leakey. "Our anterior teeth are not suited for tearing flesh or hide. We don't have large canine teeth, and we wouldn't have been able to deal with food sources that required those large canines."

Until about two and a half million years ago, we had no stone tools. The sharp canine teeth some other primates use to occasionally kill and eat small mammals had been lost to our species by at least three and a half million years ago.

"It certainly is distinctive that the hominids don't have sharp, projective canines, and the non-hominids do," Leakey said. "When you go back to three or three and a half million years, there were some hominids with canines that were perhaps marginally larger than the modern human's, but it's not a significant difference. You've got to go further back to find the origin of that adaptation. The loss of projecting canines must relate to an adaptation of some kind. I don't think they'd just disappear."

Getting rid of large canine teeth allowed our ancestors to eat the available foods more easily. Vegetation was everywhere, and food processors and cooking equipment were not yet on the scene. So we ate a great deal of plants which were uncooked. Like cattle, horses, or other vegetarians, we needed molars for crushing food rather than knife-like incisors for cutting through flesh. Without the restriction of large canine teeth, our jaws were able to move somewhat side-to-side to crush vegetation.

> *"Molecular biologists and geneticists have established very convincingly that we are closer to the chimpanzee than a horse is to a donkey. We are extraordinarily similar."*
>
> **Dr. Richard Leakey**

"If you've got interlocking canines and third molars and you close your mouth, you're basically locking it anteriorly," Leakey said. "But if you've got smaller canines that don't lock anteriorly, you've got a far greater lateral movement. There could be some benefit from reducing the size of the canines and being able to chew foods differently."

Stone Tools and Scavenging

So presumably we were eating a diet that was more in line with the essentially vegetarian non-human primates on the savannah. Then, about two-and-a-half million years ago, crude stone tools made their first appearance. We still relied on fruits and other vegetation we could pick with our hands. But with stone tools we were able to cut apart a carcass if we got a hold of one. That, of course, was another matter. We were not quick like lions or tigers. Nor were we particularly strong. Our weapons were quite crude, and hunting was very inefficient. And why bother, anyway, in a land filled with fruits and lush vegetation? The beginning of meat-eating was probably not hunting at all. It was scavenging. In times of drought, when vegetation was scarce, we may have been forced to eat the left-overs of carnivores' prey.

"If you faced a narrowing of your dietary base because of environmental change of some kind—desiccation, whatever," Leakey said, "then the only way to maintain yourself would be to change your feeding strategy. One of the options seems to have been to increase the amount of meat. Now the only way to do that is to get hold of it. If you're a bipedal primate and not particularly intelligent, the obvious way to do it is to scavenge. I mean, scavenging doesn't take a great deal of smarts. You've got to be fairly careful what you scavenge from, but in Africa on the savannah, there is invariably a lot of wasted meat on the remains. There is a wide range of scavengers: hyenas and jackals, birds, insects, and reptiles. It seems to me that a perfectly sensible new strategy is to scavenge for a while, taking from the remains of animals killed by more successful hunters—lions or other large carnivores."

Early humans, who would have had trouble catching and killing prey on their own, occasionally found left-overs waiting for them. "Lions never eat everything," Leakey said. "Lions leave anything from 10 percent to 80 percent of what they kill. Now there's quite a long line of different scavengers that have their own hierarchy, if you like, but a bipedal primate could quite easily move into that hierarchy without too much threat. I don't think that would have taken much to learn. But you're only going to be able to do that when you can cut the meat. The hyenas and vultures have got sharp equipment of their own, and you've got to be able to get at it yourself if you're going to compete with them."

The analysis of ancient animal bones supports the scavenging hypothesis. Patterns of scratches on these bones have revealed that stone tools were scraped over the bones after carnivorous teeth had cut into them, suggesting that the bones had been carnivores' prey which were then scraped clean by human scavengers.

The possibility of using stone tools to cut carcasses demanded degrees of reasoning and manipulation that had not previously occurred. It also demanded cultural changes as a new food source was exploited. "About two and a half million years ago, you suddenly find evidence of tools: sharp stones, stones that have been broken and have sharp edges," Leakey said. "These are invariably associated with bones of animals, suggesting meat in the diet in one form or another. That evidence coincides with the first appearance of an enlarged and modified brain shape. That process of cutting meat required a degree of mental equipment that was perhaps an advance over the primitive ancestral condition."

In the process, there were some unforeseen dangers of including meat in the diet, and evidently some serious mistakes, such as eating carnivore liver. The livers of carnivorous

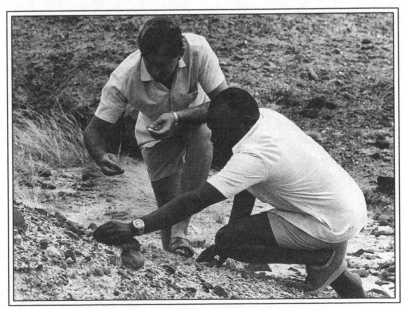

Dr. Richard Leakey and Mr. Kamoya Kimew

animals can accumulate very large concentrations of vitamin A, concentrations which could be poisonous if eaten. But early hunters did not know that. Leakey found a skeleton of an unfortunate individual whose bones showed the signs of an overdose of vitamin A.[1] Over time, humans have learned to generally avoid eating carnivores.

Of course, there are other hazards of meat-eating. Humans, as a primate species, are biologically distant from the true carnivores (e.g. feline species). We do not have a good means of handling the fat and cholesterol of meat, which routinely cause atherosclerosis, often to a fatal degree. In addition, the colon of a true carnivore is much shorter than the human colon, so that the breakdown products of meat can be rapidly eliminated. In humans, our longer colon may develop cancer when a high-fiber vegetable diet is exchanged for a high-fat meat diet. Eating meat made sense when little else was available. But the human body has never adapted to a diet that includes regular quantities of meat.

Some may imagine that early humans were essentially full-time hunters who ate nothing but meat. But the evidence does not support this idea. "Remember that the eating of meat on the African savannah," Leakey said, "although it's in big packages and you can share it, still accounts for a relatively small part of your diet. Even with the successful scavengers and successful hunters, meat is a rather small part of the diet, except in places like the Arctic, where in certain seasons meat is the only thing you can eat because there's nothing else to gather. But we are not carnivores and never have been carnivores, and that should be remembered. Some have become in modern times increasingly carnivorous because of the ready availability of meat from domestic animals. The excess of meat and the imbalance of the contemporary diet as a result of the domestication of cattle, sheep and goats, pigs, chickens, and fish, is, of course, something unusual."

Hunting and Aggression

Cave paintings depict scenes of hunts. A history of hunting, real or imagined, might imply that earliest man had a certain amount of innate aggression that nowadays translates into wars and other forms of violence. Leakey disagrees. "A predator-prey relationship is a totally different thing from individual aggression where food is not its purpose. When you go off and kill a mammoth or kill a grasshopper, one is doing it because one's hungry. The urban violence, the interpersonal violence, the international violence, and other forms of violence that so characterize contemporary times have absolutely no relationship to a hunting past. It reflects a total misunderstanding of the hunting urge, if there is such a thing as a hunting urge."

Hunting in modern times, Leakey contends, has nothing to do with survival either. "That men, in particular, find great satisfaction in hunting and in showing their bravado has all to do with our hormones and our need to display. It is a male characteristic to display prowess in an area that attracts attention both from other males and presumably from breeding females. I think what we're seeing with these chaps who go off with great guns and shoot animals that really can't do them any harm is related to a breeding strategy, a sort of macho reproductive mating dance."

> *"Forms of violence that so characterize contemporary times have absolutely no relationship to a hunting past. It reflects a total misunderstanding of the hunting urge, if there is such a thing as a hunting urge."*
>
> Dr. Richard Leakey

Evidence indicates that our species evolved mainly on a high-fiber diet of foods from plants. With little meat and no dairy products until relatively recently in the evolutionary process, fat and cholesterol would have made a much more modest contribution to our diet than they do today. It has become more and more clear that a return to the diet of our evolutionary past would be of great benefit. Just as medical research shows that meat-eating is responsible for an increase in risk of cancer, heart disease, and other illness, anthropological research has shown that our bodies were designed for an herbivorous menu. Adaptation to a new diet is a slow process. While we dine on twentieth century food, our bodies are made for quite a different diet indeed.

Chapter 9

Lessons from Asia

In their search for an optimal diet, researchers have looked for groups of people who tend to stay healthy into advanced age. Of course, no country has a perfect diet or perfect health. But Asian countries do a much better job of holding cancer, heart disease, and many other serious conditions at arm's length than do Western countries.

China has provided, in a sense, a natural laboratory. Diets vary significantly from one part of the country to another, and people tend to stay in the same place all their lives, allowing relationships between diet and health to emerge.

Most nutrition researchers have ignored this opportunity. They have focused on single nutrients such as beta-carotene, vitamin C, fiber, or any one of the hundreds of others teased out of foods, and studied them in isolation. They study whether cigarette-smokers are healthier if they take a beta-carotene pill or whether meat-eaters do better with fiber supplements, consuming vast sums of money and yielding results that are often vague or conflicting.

T. Colin Campbell and his colleagues, Chen Junshi and Li Junyao of Beijing, China, and Richard Peto of Oxford University, tried a radically different approach. In one of the most ambitious nutrition research projects ever conducted, they exploited the natural dietary variations in China. They asked, not whether one or another vitamin supplement helps, but rather, what are the health effects that come from much more comprehensive differences in the diet.

Beginning in 1983, the team collected information about the typical foods of 65 Chinese provinces. They studied records of health and illness, and took blood samples and made other tests. In 1991, they published an 896-page monograph filled with their data, which they continue to analyze, along with the results of their subsequent and even larger studies. Their first findings were that, overall, Chinese diets are extraordinarily healthy by Western standards. Rice and other grains, vegetables, and legumes are consumed in much greater quantity than in the U.S. So while Americans get 37 percent of their calories from fat, the Chinese do far better. "Fat intake in China ranges from a low of 6% of calories to a high of 24%," Campbell said. "These are average numbers for counties, so some individuals might be lower than 6% and higher than 24%. The overall average fat intake is 14.5%."

And because the diet is plant-based, it avoids most of the ill effects that come from animal protein in Western diets. "Protein intake in China, on average, is about two-thirds of what it is in the West," Campbell said. "And the kind of protein that is consumed is very different. Only about 10% of the total protein intake is from animal sources, whereas here it is about 70%. As a percent of total calories, animal protein intake is about ten times higher here than in rural China."

The Power of a Plant-Based Diet

But even though their diets are better overall, there is a range of diets within China, which allows their effect on disease rates to be studied in detail. Dietary differences result in a range of cholesterol levels and marked differences in the rates of illness. "When we look at disease rates, it becomes very clear that the lower the blood cholesterol level the better," Campbell said. "We see no evidence of a threshold of decreasing blood

"In other words, the more the diet is composed of foods of plant origin, the better it is. There appears to be no threshold."

Dr. T. Colin Campbell

cholesterol levels insofar as an association with lower chronic diseases is concerned. It also looks like the lower the fat intake the better; again there is no threshold. And the higher the fiber intake the better. In other words, the more the diet is composed of foods of plant origin, the better it is. There appears to be no threshold of plant food enrichment."

The China Study suggests that a diet composed entirely of grains, vegetables, legumes, and fruits is superior to diets containing even small amounts of meat, poultry, or other animal products. "When only a small amount of animal products are added to the diet, up to 20% of total protein or so, it makes a significant difference," Campbell said. "When we compare people on diets that are virtually nil in animal protein with those for whom animal protein is upwards of twenty to thirty percent of the total protein intake, the cholesterol levels go from around 90 milligrams per deciliter to about 170 milligrams per deciliter. And these increases in cholesterol are associated with the emergence of the cancers and heart disease that are common in the West."

Recognition of the power of plant-based diets was quite a turn-around in Campbell's own life. "I was raised on a dairy farm," Campbell said. "I milked cows from the time I was five until I was twenty-one. We had our own garden and our own livestock for meat and dairy. When I went away to school, I eventually got my Ph.D. at Cornell in animal nutrition. I worked on a project to see how we might be able to produce animal protein more efficiently. So both my personal life as well as my professional life were entirely on the other end of the research findings that we've been getting."

> *"Nutrition is a powerful regulator of the emergence of these kinds of diseases, so much so that when nutrient intakes are correct, they can virtually control the expression of these genes, no matter how risky they may be."*
>
> **Dr. T. Colin Campbell**

Of course, diet is not the only factor affecting health. Some people are exposed to toxic chemicals or other risks. Genetics plays a role. But Campbell argues that even in the presence of such risks, an optimal diet, that is, a purely plant-based diet, provides a large measure of protection.

"The question which future research needs to ask is how effective can a diet be in preventing disease among individuals who are highly susceptible either because of genes from their parents or because of their genes being altered by exposure to chemical or viral carcinogens. In other words, is it possible to prevent disease when these people consume an otherwise perfect diet? I suggest that we will eventually find that it will be possible to achieve prevention for the vast majority of people, regardless of their genetic susceptibility. Nutrition is a powerful regulator of the emergence of these kinds of diseases, so much so that when nutrient intakes are correct, they can virtually control the expression of these genes, no matter how risky they may be.

"If we consider the so-called migrant studies, we find that people who move from one area of the world to another generally take on the risk of disease of the adopted country, regardless of their presumed susceptibilities. This is a very exciting proposition because it suggests that people are not necessarily condemned by their family history."

Problems With Animal Protein

The China Study has highlighted particular risks from animal protein. Most people, of course, are more concerned about fat, because fat increases cholesterol and increases cancer risk. Should we be concerned about problems from too much protein?

"Definitely," Campbell said. "There is strong evidence in the scientific literature that when a reduction in fat is compared to a reduction in protein intake, the protein effect on blood cholesterol is more significant than the effect of saturated fat. Animal protein is a hypercholesterolemic agent. We can reduce cholesterol levels either by reducing animal protein intake or exchanging it for plant protein. Some of the plant proteins, particularly soy, have an impressive ability to reduce cholesterol. I really think that protein—both the kind and the amount—is more significant as far as cholesterol levels are concerned than is saturated fat, and certainly more significant than dietary cholesterol itself."

The reason for animal protein's dangerous effect on cholesterol is not entirely clear, but some clues have emerged.

"We do know that the consumption of animal protein has a profound effect on enzymes that are involved in the metabolism of cholesterol and related chemicals," Campbell said. "This occurs very quickly—within hours after the consumption of the meal. "Whether it is the immune system, various enzyme systems, the uptake of carcinogens into the cells, or hormonal activities, animal protein generally only causes mischief. High fat intake still can be a problem, and we ought not to be consuming such high-fat diets. But I suggest that animal protein is more problematic in this whole diet/disease relationship than is total fat."

> *"Whether it is the immune system, various enzyme systems, the uptake of carcinogens into the cells, or hormonal activities, animal protein generally only causes mischief."*
>
> **Dr. T. Colin Campbell**

Of course, in the very recent past, animal protein was regarded as a healthful, if not essential, source of nutrition. The result has been reluctance to consider possible health risks of animal protein and advantages of plant protein. "Protein is a nutrient that is so highly regarded by everyone, including investigators themselves, that there is a tremendous bias against considering its ability to control disease," Campbell said. "It is easy to see that fat is greasy and nasty, so most people more readily accept the idea that fat might have something to do with the emergence of disease. They do not want to imagine that animal protein does the same thing as excess fat intake. But it turns out that animal protein, when consumed, exhibits a variety of undesirable health effects."

The result is that Westerners tend to prefer to switch from one animal protein source to another, such as from beef to chicken breast, rather than to plant-based diets. Yet a switch from beef to poultry is not likely to help much, if at all. "The existing evidence suggests that this makes little or no sense," Campbell said. "It may reduce fat intake a bit, but even lean cuts of meat or poultry still contain around 20-40% of total calories as fat, or even more. This is not going to get us very far. It might get our fat intake down a bit, but our protein intake is not going to change; if anything its already high level may go even higher. One really has to change the total diet. Anything less than that is a cruel hoax on the population at large. It doesn't make sense."

The Women's Health Trial feasibility study was a case in point. It was a three-year trial which found that women will, in fact, follow dietary advice they are offered. But the focus was only on reducing fat intake. They did reduce their fat intake from 37 percent of calories to 23 percent. But reductions in "red meat" were in large measure counterbalanced by increases in poultry and fish, with no improvement in the consumption of grains, vegetables, and legumes.[1]

One would not expect to see good results from such a change, and, in fact, studies have shown that modest reductions in fat intake have no effect on breast cancer rates,[2] and only a very modest effect on other illnesses.

Likewise, the China Study does not suggest that supplements of beta-carotene or vitamin C are any substitute for major dietary changes. "These cosmetic changes—taking out a little fat or adding some supposedly protective nutrients— are not going to achieve the results that we all think are possible," Campbell said. "We might see reduction in some diseases with the use of supplements, but that is such an unpredictable response, and we tend not to take into consideration the down side of using those supplements during the long term. Taking supplements as a means of preventing or treating these diseases is a very superficial approach. It just simply is not the nutritional way to reduce disease."

> *"One really has to change the total diet. Anything less than that is a cruel hoax on the population at large. It doesn't make sense."*
>
> *Dr. T. Colin Campbell*

A 1994 study of 29,000 smokers in Finland showed that beta-carotene or vitamin E pills did nothing to reduce their risk of lung cancer. In fact, those taking beta-carotene supplements actually had a higher incidence of lung cancer than those taking a placebo.[3]

The good news is that more profound dietary changes exert much more profound effects on health. Campbell found, for example, that diet appears to affect hormone function, which in turn, influences the age of puberty and other factors.

"Menarche—a girl's first period—starts between fifteen and nineteen years of age in China, whereas it is twelve to thirteen in the United States," Campbell said. "As you know, a later age of menarche is correlated with a lower rate of breast cancer, at least when comparing different populations. So this later age of menarche in China is indicative of disease prevention in a sense."

What causes the difference in the age of puberty? The onset of puberty is triggered when a girl reaches a certain point in her growth. If she is on a high-fat, low-fiber diet that accelerates growth, she will have an early puberty and a higher risk of breast cancer later in life. "Of course, that is also the kind of diet that tends to elevate circulating estrogen levels," Campbell said. "So I think a lot of breast cancer could be accounted for by an overly rapid early growth rate in the United States. Now, this doesn't mean that we can't bring breast cancer under control later in life. For women who grew fast in the beginning, the evidence suggests that, were they to change their diets later on in life, they should be able to set back the inevitable progression to breast cancer."

The Chinese have a different experience at the beginning of their reproductive years. They also have a very different experience at menopause, as Campbell points out. "Chinese physicians who have worked with me say there are less problems at that age than there appear to be in the West. One hypothesis, if this is true, is that, in the case of Western women where the estrogen levels are sustained at fairly high levels throughout their reproductive years because of their high-fat diets, when they reach menopause those estrogen levels drop precipitously to the natural baseline levels. For women on lower-fat diets, these circulating estrogen levels are somewhat lower during the reproductive years, so they don't drop so markedly at menopause. The more rapid drop that we see in Western women may put them at higher risk for the adverse effects associated with metabolic adjustment, such as with calcium loss, for example."

The benefits of lower-fat diets, then, are not just fewer problems with hot flashes and mood swings. There are also 80 percent fewer hip fractures in China, compared to Western countries.

Westerners can take advantage of the benefits of plant-based diets themselves. Adapting is much easier than many people might imagine, as Campbell found out in his own family. "We started changing our diet when our children came along, and we have been changing ever since. I really don't see that a change, if desired, is that big of a deal. In the short run, people who are accustomed to a high-salt, high-fat diet are not going to like healthier foods at first. But if they have a little patience, they will find that after two or three months, perhaps longer, they adapt to new tastes. And then they discover new tastes that they never realized were there before."

From Prevention to Treatment

Asian traditions have contributed to our knowledge of how dietary changes help prevent illness. They have also provided novel treatments. One of the best known examples comes from Anthony Sattilaro, M.D., who was the President of Methodist Hospital in Philadelphia. In 1978, Dr. Sattilaro was diagnosed with prostate cancer. In older men, prostate cancer often follows a very slow course. But in younger men, like Dr. Sattilaro, prostate cancer is a grave disease. Modern medicine has done little to change the prognosis. When Dr. Sattilaro was found to have prostate cancer that had spread throughout his body, he was told to prepare for his death.

I met Dr. Sattilaro almost 10 years later, in 1986. Not only was he alive; he was youthful and vigorous. His cancer was gone, so far as his doctors could tell, and foods seemed to have played a major role in the change. And, a bit later on, other foods may have played a very malignant role. But first, the beginning of the story.

"I became the President of Methodist Hospital in 1977," Sattilaro said. "In May of 1978, in between all kinds of meetings with planners and builders, I went for my annual physical. A chest X-ray was routine at that time. About an hour after I got back to my office, I got a call from radiology.

"The radiologist said, 'How do you feel?' I said, 'I feel well. I'm too busy to be sick.' He said, 'You've got something in your left lung.' So I walked to the second floor to the radiology department, and sure enough, there was a golf-ball-sized lesion in the left lung. He thought it was in the lung, but said it might be in the rib. We then did a bone scan, which showed lesions in three areas of the skull, the right shoulder, two vertebrae, the entire sternum, and the left sixth rib.

"This was *not* in the program for the day. It wasn't on the calendar. It was such a crashing experience, realizing that your whole world was coming to an end. Cancer, to me, was a death sentence. Nothing was in perspective anymore. The biopsy results showed prostate cancer with metastases."

The cancer had begun in the prostate, but had metastasized, that is spread, to his bones. The result is often severe pain as the cancer grows within the bone.

"Cancer of the prostate in patients under 50 is a terminal disease. There are no survivors. After 50, the disease is very different. I had seen any number of patients who were 75 or 80 who had cancers of the prostate which were relatively benign.

"I knew the surgeon very well, and I also happened to be going to an internist who, by chance, was an oncologist and a good friend. I was told, literally, to get my affairs in order. I wasn't prepared to do that. I had just turned 48. The question was, why me? This is wrong. I went through that kind of agonizing, without much spiritual support, nothing to hold onto, and with all of the scientific data saying you're going to die and you have to get ready to do that. And I did. I put all of my affairs in order.

"I went back to work quickly. Work was a placebo for the pain. But I was then taking large doses of narcotics, and they finally put me on a thing called Brompton's mixture, which is morphine, cocaine, and Compazine. It's used in hospices. The morphine gave you a euphoria, but made you very nauseated, so the Compazine cut the vomiting down. The cocaine gave you an 'up' for the 'down' you get after the morphine. With the help of my assistant, I was able to block out interviews. I would wait until my speech wasn't slurred, and I'd be able to look as though I was operating pretty well.

"Then my father died with terminal cancer throughout his body. He died at Methodist Hospital. We went to the burial plot in central New Jersey, right near the little town where I had grown up. My mother was there, and we buried him on the seventh of August.

"Afterward, I got on the New Jersey Turnpike. It was beastly hot. There were two hitchhikers, and I picked them up. One fell asleep in the back seat. The other one was named Sean McLean, and we got to talking. I told him about the sad event I had just experienced, my father's death, and that I was dying, that I was going to be dead in a year or so. And he said very glibly to me, which annoyed the hell out of me, 'You don't have to die, Doc, cancer's easy to cure.'

"First of all, that's a very adolescent response to this great doctor, who knows that cancer isn't easy to cure. Here was somebody, a guy who was a cook, certainly not in my educational class, saying by absolute faith that it was easy to cure. And I have to say that I just dismissed him. He had graduated from cooking school, and he and his friend were going to South Carolina for a holiday before going to work. But something made him hook on to me. He said, 'We'll get off with you in Philadelphia. We're going to take you to a natural foods store.' Well, that was the last thing I was interested in. I have never had any real interest in food, and to this day I don't, except from what's happened to me. Meals were always very quick.

"So we went to the natural foods store, and I was utterly repelled by it. I thought natural foods were for people who just couldn't afford to eat meat and that they were all strange people who were against the Vietnam war and so on. I had the wildest ideas about vegetarians and people who ate natural foods.

"I went back to the hospital and I proceeded to do my work. Then about two weeks later I got a whole packet of information from these guys, with 67 cents postage due. It was about macrobiotics. Well, I looked at it and it was just pure garbage to me. The whole series of anecdotal stories saying 'I ate this way, and I did A, B, C, D, E and I got well.' You and I have seen that for any kind of thing. Vitamin C does it, or my trip with yoga does it, or all sorts of things. But something caught my eye. There was a physician who gave a testimonial. It was articulately done, and she was living in Philadelphia. So, I said, what the hell. It's my dime. I'll just call her.

"I remember the night very clearly. Her husband answered. I told him who I was, and I said, 'Tell me about your wife. She claims that she's had some really good results with this macrobiotic stuff.' And he said, 'Oh Doc, she's marvelous when she eats that way, but she hates the food. And she's now dying of cancer in the hospital. She can't eat that way.'

"She had abandoned the diet. I got intrigued by his very firm belief that diet was instrumental in her breast cancer. Here was a hormonally sensitive tumor of the breast, and I had prostate cancer, which is also hormone-related. And for whatever reasons, I guess it was a combination of pain, desperation, desolation, and just not wanting to die, I then decided that I would pursue the macrobiotic thing.

"I looked up the macrobiotic people in Philadelphia. And that was a vision to behold. I went to their house. I had to take my shoes off. And I sat down in the study of this very Asian-looking house on the outskirts of Philadelphia. This young fellow looked at my face, and looked at my eyes, and diagnosed my cancer using Asian methods, which I have learned since. He said, 'We can get you well.' And he wanted me to start on this very rigid diet, and I said, 'Well, I can't, I'm going to Italy next week.' He said, 'I beg you not to leave the United States. This is very important. You must get on this diet.' Well, I said okay.

"His wife gave me a cooking lesson on Saturday. I went out to buy this stuff, and it was just a complete blunder. First of all, I'd never been in the kitchen. I come from an Italian family where men never went into the kitchen. So I didn't know how to turn the stove on. To this day, I'm still clumsy in the kitchen. And I blew up the pot of brown rice. It was just a mess. An absolute mess. And I sat down and cried.

"So, I talked to them, and they were really nice. They said 'Well, why don't you come and eat with us? You can take your lunch to the hospital.' Well, I didn't know what I was getting into. It was a real community, a commune. The first night I went there, it seemed very strange, sitting on the floor and eating with chopsticks.

"But it was a challenge to me, because as I sat and listened to his lectures, everything that he was talking about was completely the opposite of what I had been taught. He taught me the five-element theory of diagnosis, how we interplay with nature, and the unified theory of disease. None of those things had ever been part of my medical training. We talked about problems with lungs, problems with kidneys, and so forth. They believe that there is an intermingling of all of these systems. It took me a long time to come to grips with that and then start realizing that it worked. Nobody at the hospital minded much, because I wasn't doing anything but bringing my food in. People were mostly sympathetic. They said, well, he's dying. What the hell. We'll kind of support somebody who's dying.

"Then I started taking it seriously for a couple of reasons. Three weeks after I started the diet, I was able to throw all of the drugs away. I didn't have to take any more morphine. The pain disappeared. When you have chronic pain, to get a day free, you'd have conversations with the devil. That's how debilitating pain is.

"Well, that was the first step. I stayed in the community, although the people there were entirely different from me. They were 25 years younger than I was, with a whole set of values that was totally different, living very simple lives, eating food that had virtually no taste to it, forcing me to chew everything a hundred times. I could not say that I enjoyed the food at all, but I couldn't argue with the fact that I was feeling better.

"I took a trip to Puerto Rico in November of that year. I got to Puerto Rico and went off the diet one day. I had bouillabaisse, fish soup. The next morning I was terribly sick. I turned around and left Puerto Rico and came back to Philadelphia. I remember just the loneliest Thanksgiving that I've ever had in my life, because the macrobiotic household was closed. I went to a Japanese restaurant and was the only person in the restaurant.

"My mother was very supportive. She was also very depressed. My father had just died, and so it was a very difficult time for her. And I couldn't help her with that, because I was dealing with my own collapse. I couldn't handle

> *"Then I started taking it [macrobiotics] seriously for a couple of reasons. Three weeks after I started the diet, I was able to throw all of the drugs away."*
>
> **Dr. Anthony Sattilaro**

my father's death, either, and I couldn't handle her emotions. I couldn't support her.

"The remarkable thing about all of this was that I started getting better. By winter, when I was supposed to be going downhill, my hemoglobin levels were going up. I was feeling better; I had increased energy. By Easter time, I was back to my old self. And nobody could believe it.

"Well, it was the late spring, and I said to my oncologist, 'I'm not a fool. I think there's a lot of quackery that I'm involved in here. But there's something to this dietary approach.' He said, 'Tony, come on, we know what's going on here. You're one of those people who's doing better than we had expected.'

> *"The remarkable thing about all of this was that I started getting better. By winter, when I was supposed to be going downhill, my hemoglobin levels were going up. And nobody could believe it."*
>
> **Dr. Anthony Sattilaro**

"Then September came, and I had my annual X-ray. We took the X-ray, and that made history. Here was a case of a person who had had documented cancer, who had some things go radically differently in his life. The cancer was gone.

"Well, that was enough for me to start dealing with my cynicism. I still could not accept the society that I had been drawn into, because it was totally foreign to me. But I had to give credence to the fact that maybe there was something here.

"Things were going well at the hospital. It was building and growing. People were excited that I was well, although not very excited that I was eating a loony kind of diet and bringing chopsticks in, but I did it all with a sense of humor. That was the time when it was brought out that humor has an effect on disease. I treated it all as a big game. I just made up my mind that I would get well and went along with the whole show.

"So, in my private life I became a classical macrobiotic doing everything, including sleeping on a futon, having a gas stove in my apartment, and never wearing any synthetic clothes; everything was cotton. It was a 180-degree switch. Then I met Jean Kohler, who was a musicologist who had had pancreatic cancer. He wrote *Healing Miracles Through*

Macrobiotics. I read that book, and I was inspired by talking to him and to his wife on the phone. His cancer had disappeared, and he attributed it to the diet. So I stayed on it and got very involved with the macrobiotic community. And the more I read, the more I became seduced by the whole concept that everything was upside down in the West, that we were starting from the wrong side."

Sattilaro looked and felt terrific. He began to write of his experiences and to give lectures to audiences seeking the same cure he had apparently found. He felt so good, in fact, that he was tempted to believe he no longer needed the diet he was on. "I had thought about quitting," he said, "simply because I was now well. And what the hell, why did I need to do it any more? But they made it very clear that the cancer would come back and warned me that if it should come back, it would be very hard to cure it a second time. So I was terrified and, at the same time, seduced by the whole thing.

"Then I had to face the reality of what was going on. Was this an 'unexplained remission?' That's what we say in science when we don't understand something. There are some people who can get a deadly cancer and then for some reason or other it goes

> *"Here was a case of a person who had had documented cancer, who had some things go radically differently in his life. The cancer was gone."*
>
> **Dr. Anthony Sattilaro**

away. We know that we can change what happens to our blood vessels. Those data are all in. Can we change what happens with cancer? My answer is unequivocally yes. I think we can not only prevent cancer; I believe that we can cure cancer. But I don't believe that we can cure cancer after we've taken a patient and put him through a horrible series of treatments that debilitates the normal response to cancer. Now, I'm not suggesting that we stop using chemicals. There are cancers that respond well and some cancers that respond to surgery. Fine. But if you're giving people stuff simply because they want it, or because you don't know what else to do, my answer is, why not look at alternatives? I don't think they're all quackery.

"It's eight years now. Why hasn't the cancer come back? They never took the cancer out. The cancer's still in the prostate. They don't feel it. Why did it go into remission? Where is it?

"It's fine for oncologists to say this is an unexplained remission. I think it's more responsible to explain the remission. We can't just simply laugh it off. After all, if I am a case that did get well with all these variables, why not use those variables in a lot of people? It would be terrific to test it. There are enough data now to show that certain types of cancer occur with less frequency among vegetarians. Seventh-day Adventists are a classic example of that. People who live in Asia are classic examples of that. And now we're able to collect pretty good data from Asia. I think it would be good to test it. Certainly for prevention. As a cure? I used it as a cure. Whether it cured me or not, I have no idea."

In spite of his experiences, Dr. Sattilaro never rejected Western medicine. As a physician trained in diagnosis and treatment, and as an administrator of a major metropolitan hospital which had helped a great many people, he saw the value of the Western medical tradition. Eastern medicine should be added to it, not used to simply replace it. "No way. We have Western minds. We have a system of thinking called logic that's got an Aristotelian base. But we also can't dismiss all of that knowledge of the East. The East is a complement to what we have in the West.

"The first step, obviously, is to get rid of the high-fat diet and go to high-fiber. Ten years ago, this was considered a radical idea. Now look at the television commercials with all the cereals competing. Of course, that's not the answer. It's a step. It's certainly better than ham and eggs."

A macrobiotic diet is a dramatic shift from a standard American diet. Its foods come from Asian culinary traditions, and explanations of its effect are derived from ancient Chinese medical concepts. So Western doctors and laypersons alike need a bit of effort to come to grips with it.

"When I went into macrobiotics, I didn't do it because I wanted to," Sattilaro said. "I had no choice. I don't think that an American public that doesn't know it's ill, and particularly a physician public that doesn't know how food affects the body, is anywhere near ready to make that kind of a leap. It takes a lot of energy and effort, because it is a life-style change, and I don't think most Americans want a life-style change. We are now addicted to the method, 'Doctor, get me well.' And doctor does get somebody well in many diseases."

Perhaps that is part of the reason Dr. Sattilaro finally did drop the diet. In spite of his own acknowledgment that abandoning the diet might cause the return of the cancer, he took that risk. "In the last three years, I haven't done macrobiotics. I went off the diet deliberately three years ago, to test the hypothesis that vegetarianism alone would still sustain me. I slowly went to a balanced vegetarian diet that included fish. Then I added chicken to the diet. I had three years of nonmacrobiotics to compare with five years of macrobiotics. And there was no cancer."

However, emerging health problems made him return to the macrobiotic diet, after his three-year experiment with more permissive diets.

"I've gone back," he said. "That experiment's over, because of the edema, the swelling, that I have in my hands. I'm going to try the macrobiotic approach to get my whole system back in balance."

But he did not get back in balance. As he had previously predicted, his cancer returned. In July, 1989, I spoke to him for the last time. He had resumed the use of pain-killers, which at times caused him to become quite groggy. He knew that the end was near.

Dr. Sattilaro was never sure that the regimen he followed could take credit for his decade-long reprieve from cancer. Nor do we know whether, had he not deviated from the diet, first to fish, then to chicken, he would have been able to keep his cancer at bay.

But it is clear that humble foods from the plant kingdom have enormous power, both to prevent disease and to alter its course—power that we have barely begun to tap. There are many variations on healthful diets, from diets based mainly on raw foods, to macrobiotic menus drawn from traditional Asian cuisine, to diets including the full range of vegetarian foods.

It is my hope that the wealth of knowledge and experience presented by the experts in this volume will illuminate much of what is already known about the power of foods and will intrigue the reader to explore those areas which are only beginning to be understood.

Chapter 10

Recommendations

The world of nutrition is getting simpler. The same food choices that trim cholesterol levels also help trim the waistline. The menu that helps hold cancer at bay also helps prevent gallstones and problems as seemingly remote as hemorrhoids and varicose veins.

This chapter is a prescription for an optimal menu. All of the experts in this book have their own recommendations, which vary a bit from one another depending on their individual experiences and their reading of the scientific literature. But there are clear trends which are common to all. What follows are recommendations for a most potent regimen for health.

There are two main principles:

1. Shift from animal sources to plant foods.
2. Shift from refined foods to unrefined foods.

Animal sources are too high in fat, protein, and contaminants, and leave out fiber and carbohydrate. They always contain cholesterol, while foods from plants never contain cholesterol. Foods from animals never contain fiber; all fiber comes from plants. Meats also contain a generous portion of saturated fat, which stimulates the body to make cholesterol. No meats are as low in fat as typical grains, beans, vegetables, and fruits.

Refining has added to our problems. Refined flours leave out much of the fiber. Sugars are products of refining which leaves out the other plant components. Vegetable oils can also be considered a refined product, in the sense that the oil is extracted from a plant and used in a concentrated form. Oil is a natural part of corn, soybeans, olives, nuts, and other plant foods. When oils are extracted and used in pure form, the diet begins to contain too much oil. Picture the chimpanzees' diet. The fiber was not extracted. Oil was consumed only as an intrinsic part of plants.

Foods to Include

The principal foods that make up a healthy diet are these:

◆ *Grains* are packed with fiber, and have a healthful blend of carbohydrates, protein, vitamins, and minerals, and just a trace of fat. Include generous amounts of whole grain breads, pasta, cereals, and rice in your daily routine.

◆ *Legumes* (beans, lentils, etc.) come in endless varieties. Many are identified with particular cultures such as pinto beans in the American Southwest, black beans in Mexico's Yucatan peninsula, or navy beans in England and, of course, in Boston. Beans are excellent sources of fiber, protein, carbohydrates, iron, and calcium.

◆ *Vegetables* come in many varieties and are packed with vitamins and minerals. Include several generous portions each day.

◆ *Fruits* contain more than the vitamin C they are famous for. They contain other vitamins, minerals, and certain kinds of fiber, as well. As the favorite food of our primate cousins, we should bring fruits back onto the menu.

Nuts, nut butters, and seeds should not be a large part of the diet. They are rich in minerals, but should be used sparingly because of their high fat content.

Foods to Exclude

◆ *"Red Meat:"* Actor James Garner appeared in commercials for the beef industry, calling beef "real food for real people." But as the ads were airing, Garner was hospitalized for a coronary bypass and a dissecting aneurysm of his aorta—the main artery of the body was literally tearing apart. Happily, Garner recovered. He changed his diet and switched to doing car commercials. The moral of the story is that if you're a "real person" eating that kind of "real food," you should live real close to a real good hospital, because you are likely to have very real problems. Meat contains too much fat and cholesterol and provides nothing that we cannot get from more healthful sources. Castelli, DeBakey, and virtually all other experts in coronary disease recommend reducing the amount of meat in the diet. How much should it be reduced? Castelli says that the best diet contains no meat at all.

◆ *Poultry and Fish:* Rosenthal and McDougall may have surprised some readers by pointing out that poultry is not exactly a health food. First of all, poultry contains no fiber whatsoever. Second, it contains no carbohydrate. Third, chicken contains essentially the same amount of cholesterol as beef: 25 milligrams (mg) per ounce. As Castelli pointed out, every 100 mg of cholesterol consumed on a daily basis raises serum cholesterol about five points. Chicken's undeserved reputation as a healthier food than beef stems from its usually lower fat con-tent when the skin and dark meat are discarded and a non-fat cooking method is used. But even then, chicken is still much higher in fat than grains, legumes, vegetables, and fruits and, like all meats, is devoid of fiber and carbohydrate. About a third of poultry products are contaminated with live salmonella bacteria, and residues of pesticides and other chemicals are common.

McDougall says, "I don't tell people to switch from beef and pork to chicken and fish, because it's no switch at all. They're still fiber-free and still high on the food chain of contamination. I explain to people that these are muscles. They wiggle tails and move legs, no matter which animal they come from."

Poultry, like all meats, is essentially a mixture of protein and fat. Too much fat, of course, is bad for us. But so is too much protein. When we eat too much protein, we aggravate our risk of osteoporosis, kidney disease, and possibly certain forms of cancer.

Similar concerns relate to fish. Some species of fish are lower in cholesterol and fat content than "red meats" or poultry. But fish does contain cholesterol and fat, and is devoid of fiber. Fish is concentrated in protein and contributes to osteoporosis and kidney problems. Regarding contamination, fish are easily the worst offenders because they receive almost no inspection at all and often live in polluted areas.

Because they are carnivorous, they tend to concentrate contaminants from the prey they have eaten.

◆ *Dairy Products and Eggs:* Dairy products are a peculiar invention. From a historical standpoint, these foods were only very recently made a part of human cuisine, and many cultures have not yet accepted the practices of milk consumption after weaning or the consumption of milk from animals. The dairy industry has a powerful lobby which has aggressively promoted its products. There is, however, nothing in milk which is not available in a more healthful form in other foods. As we saw in Chapter 6, green leafy vegetables and beans contain calcium without the cholesterol, fat, and allergenic proteins of dairy products. Eggs contain a whopping dose of cholesterol and far more protein than is required in anyone's diet.

◆ *Oils:* To keep our cholesterol levels low, plant oils are better than animal fats. But, in general, we should avoid added fats and oils. Whether they are saturated or unsaturated, from animals or plants, all fats and oils seem to increase cancer risk. In addition, they have more than twice the calories of either carbohydrates or proteins, ounce for ounce. Fried foods and recipes that call for added oil are the principal sources of vegetable oil. So, it is no good getting away from beef and chicken if french fries and potato chips take their place.

Special Concerns

There are three considerations that often concern people who are steering clear of meats: protein, calcium, and vitamin B-12. The first two are not problems in reality, although the third dose require some attention.

Protein

People have unfortunately come to view protein as synonymous with health. We eat it, we put it on our hair—if we were told it would make a shinier car wax, we'd probably believe it. The fact is, we do need protein in our diet. But we do not need large amounts of protein. And there are good reasons to limit high-protein foods. As Drs. McDougall and Rosenthal have explained, high-protein diets contribute to two problems: kidney disease and osteoporosis. A higher intake of protein forces the kidneys to work harder and probably to lose function earlier. Likewise, high-protein diets cause calcium to be lost in the urine. For reasons that are not entirely clear, the amino acids that are released when high-protein meals are consumed cause significant amounts of calcium to be excreted in the urine.

Since meats, poultry, and fish are simply muscles, they are basically mixtures of protein and fat, with no fiber or carbohydrate. It is virtually impossible to include significant quantities of these foods without escalating protein intake beyond desirable levels. The protein that is inherent in a varied diet of grains, vegetables, fruits, and legumes, is more than sufficient for the body's needs, and the inclusion of animal products tends to escalate protein intake to higher than desirable levels.

How much protein should be included in the diet? As a practical matter, there is no reason to get out your food scale and nutrition tables. The best rule of thumb is to have a variety of foods in sufficient quantity to maintain a reasonable body weight. It is not necessary to consciously combine various foods in order to assure adequate protein. A normally varied diet of foods from plants will provide plenty of protein. If you include meat, poultry, or fish, on a regular basis, you are almost certainly getting too much.

Calcium

There has been a considerable amount of misinformation about calcium lately, as Burkitt and others have pointed out. Although some have suggested that the calcium in milk will slow or stop the process of osteoporosis, many studies have shown little or no benefit from boosting intake of milk or calcium in general. Preventive steps include weight-bearing exercise, avoiding smoking and excessive alcohol consumption, and, as noted above, moderating protein consumption. People eating overly generous amounts of protein lose more calcium in their urine than people who have more modest protein intake.

Where is the calcium in the diet? Fortified orange juice is loaded with calcium in a form easily absorbed by the body.

Calcium supplements which contain aluminum are not recommended; neither are dairy products. Dairy products are
rich in calcium, but they contain cholesterol, fat, proteins that
can trigger allergic reactions, lactose sugar that for some
people is difficult to digest and is linked to serious health
problems, and a variety of contaminants.

Vitamin B-12

If you eliminate animal products from your diet, be sure
to include a source of vitamin B-12. B-12 is important for maintaining healthy blood and healthy nerves for people of all ages.
It is made by one-celled organisms—bacteria and algae. We
need their help in obtaining this essential vitamin. Animals,
including the human animal, cannot make vitamin B-12.

Dietary B-12 deficiencies are rare. The body carries a
several-year supply. But modern times have made deficiency
possible. In the non-industrialized world, B-12 produced by
bacteria remains on vegetables and the bacteria in manure
spread B-12 to vegetables as well. In addition, bacteria on the
teeth may also produce B-12. But the improved hygiene,
careful washing, and modern processing of the Western world
destroy the bacteria that make B-12. So Western countries
have largely lost these traditional sources of this vitamin.

Meanwhile, Westerners have gradually increased their
meat intake, which also provides a source of B-12, because,
although animals cannot make the vitamin, animals absorb
the B-12 made by bacteria which live in their digestive tracts.
This B-12 finds its way into animals' muscles, organs, and milk.

A number of people who avoid animal products have
been known to have sufficient B-12 in their bodies for years
without any apparent dietary source. Some cases of dietary B-
12 deficiency have occurred, however. There is no reason for
a deficiency, since it is very easy to include a source of the
vitamin in your routine.

Where do we find it? All common multivitamin tablets
contain B-12 and many foods, particularly breakfast cereals,
are en-riched with B-12. On labels, look for its chemical name,
"cyanocobalamin." The Recommended Daily Allowance is two
micrograms, and only about one microgram per day is actually
required.[1] B-12 tablets are commonly sold in nutrition or

"health food" stores. Fermented soy products such as miso and tempeh have been known to contain significant amounts of B-12, however only those foods produced with traditional Asian methods are likely to contain this vitamin. Western techniques for manufacture generally destroy the bacteria that produce B-12. Spirulina supplements do not contain significant amounts of true B-12.

The Process of Change

We need not adhere 100 percent to an ideal diet all the time. But change does have to be significant. Small changes are of little or no help. If weight loss, preventing cancer or heart disease, or simply staying healthy are your goals, adherence to sound dietary principles should be as close to complete as possible.

The scientific literature makes a case for a low-fat, vegetarian diet. But even many people who recognize that a meatless diet is clearly preferable are rather slow to adopt it. The reason is habit. Most of us were raised eating foods that we now know are dangerous for us. We became used to those foods, and giving them up overnight sounds like a challenge.

The following are a few suggestions for changing the menu:

1. *Take control of the kitchen.* Now that you know a great deal about healthy eating, do not let others who do not care about healthy eating dictate what you eat. Put orange traffic cones around the kitchen door and a padlock on the refrigerator. If you cook healthy foods, your family will eat them. Even though the gluttonous gene has asserted itself very strongly in the human species, people are lazier than they are gluttonous. If you have cooked something healthy, your family will eat it rather than going to the trouble of cooking something themselves.

2. *Think international.* Ethnic restaurants often have elegant meatless meals. Italian restaurants have spaghetti with tomato sauce; Mexican restaurants have bean burritos; Indian restaurants feature vegetarian curries of all kinds; Chinese restaurants have whole menu sections of vegetable entrees; Middle-Eastern restaurants feature hummus, falafel, and other delicious foods; Thai restaurants are increasingly

popular. Learning to enjoy these tastes and cooking ideas can be tremendously rewarding.

3. Enjoy the process of dietary exploration. Explore new restaurants, health-food stores, and the cookbook shelves in book stores. People love shopping. So, gratify the urge and explore new foods.

4. Find your dozen recipes. A dozen recipes is about all a family tends to use, so there is no need to be a gourmet. Simply experiment until you have found those meals that your family or friends like.

5. Be selective in fast-food choices. Most fast-food outlets are dangerous places. Avoid the burger and fried chicken routine. Many now feature generous salad bars and baked potatoes. Look for bean burritos at Mexican fast-food restaurants. To cut cholesterol at pizza outlets, ask for extra tomato sauce and all the vegetable toppings and no cheese on pizza, or spaghetti with tomato sauce. Even some burger restaurants can make meatless "burgers," which substitute lettuce, tomatoes, and toppings for meat patties.

6. Try "transition foods." Vegetarian "hot dogs," burgers, and other simulated meats help alleviate the anxiety about leaving so much cholesterol behind. Look for these at health food stores. Seventh Day Adventist food stores are a gold mine of transition foods. Take advantage of these foods during initial phases. Be careful, though—although they use vegetable oil, some contain too much of it to be permanent parts of your routine.

These and other ideas are described in more detail in Chapter 11.

As you plan your meals, be generous with grains, such as whole grain cereals, breads, brown or wild rice, and pasta. Include regular amounts of legumes, such as beans, split peas, or lentils, but don't overdo it on this rather rich protein source. Load up with vegetables; include more than one at a meal. Consider using vegetables as the focus for a meal, as in a pasta salad or with rice, rather than just as a side dish. As far as animal products and fatty foods are concerned, avoid them completely.

I hope you enjoy your explorations of new foods and the years of health they bring you.

Chapter 11

Beyond Will Power

In changing any long-standing habit, it helps to go beyond will power. Simply forcing yourself to change does not always work. There are methods that make the process of changing the menu enjoyable and rewarding. In this chapter, we will look at ways to readjust our tastes to enjoy the process of exploring new foods and to handle cravings and other problems.

First, a word about success. There is a common misperception that habits never change. And as a result, doctors are often reluctant to recommend rigorous life-style changes. So they compromise, often weakening their recommendations beyond any value.

But in 1982, Stanley Schachter of Columbia University published a study that showed something quite different. He looked at two problems: smoking and overweight.[1] He found that while people might not quit smoking the first time they try—or the second time or the third time, ultimately tremendous numbers of people *do* quit. Previous studies had mistakenly looked at whether a single *attempt* would succeed, rather than whether the *person* would succeed. Most people require more than one attempt, but before long, a great many achieve their goals. Schachter found that the same was true of weight loss. He found that many, many people have lost a great deal of weight and kept it off. Sometimes it took more than one try. But most did so without their doctors' help. So you certainly can succeed. Even though you may have had long-standing eating habits that require substantial change, you definitely can do it. And there's no time like the present to get started!

Changing Your Tastes

The first step is to change our tastes. Greasy burgers, fried chicken, gravy, ice cream, and french fries attract us like moths to a flame. When I was in college, my friends and I would routinely make late-night visits to the local "greasy spoon" cafe for "monster burgers" and onions rings, all dripping in fat. We were virtually addicted to those greasy foods.

There is a saying in science that, as individuals develop and grow, they go through stages similar to the stages the human species has gone through in its evolution. (*"Ontogeny recapitulates phylogeny."*) This seems to be true for food habits too. Early humans ate very little meat and had, instead, mainly a vegetable diet. Just as our species did not begin as carnivores, children are not born as meat-eaters. Toddlers often dislike meat at first. Unfortunately, encouragement from their well-meaning parents pushes the child's tastes toward fatty foods. The introduction of meat to children, like its introduction into cultures, radically increases the child's risk of later illness. A progressive increase in meat consumption has occurred over the last century and has led to an increase in deaths from serious illnesses. Fatty foods have established themselves in many cultures and do not seem to want to leave. Many cultures are bringing in fast-food restaurants of all kinds, but none are getting rid of them.

Happily, breaking a food habit is much easier than quitting smoking or breaking other habits. There are plenty of foods that you can substitute for less healthful ones. So let's break some habits. If you tend to spread butter or margarine on toast, on potatoes, or on vegetables, try them with less, and eventually with none at all. If you are used to a pat of butter on a baked potato, try using a half a pat. You will be surprised how quickly you can get used to less grease in your foods. Then experiment with other things in place of butter. Dijon mustard, catsup, steak sauce, Mexican sauce, or vegetables piled onto the potato can take the place of butter or margarine.

If you are a milk drinker, you should reset your taste for fat in dairy products too. When I was about 15, my mother announced that we would no longer have whole milk in the house. The skim milk she bought at first seemed watery and tasteless. But as we got used to it, whole milk began to seem much too thick and fatty, a bit like paint. Try low-fat soy or rice milks, which come in a variety of flavors. These are preferable to cow's milk for a variety of reasons, as we have seen.

Treat Yourself to the Movies

Here is a simple and fun test (for movie lovers only) that helps show how easy it is to reset your taste for fat. Treat yourself to a movie several times in the next month or two. Each time, have some popcorn with no butter or oil at all. If you are used to greasy foods, fat-free popcorn will seem bland at first. But you will soon become accustomed to the greaseless flavor. You will be, in fact, resetting your taste for fat to a lower level. Then, one time, order popcorn with the usual amount of added oil or butter. You will find the buttered variety almost intolerably greasy. When you are eating well, greasy foods become quite unattractive. By the way, if you view popcorn as a "junk food," it is not. It's a low-fat food with reasonable amounts of protein and carbohydrate. It's only when butter, oil, or salt are added that problems start.

The same phenomenon should be tried with your taste for salt. Notice that you can become accustomed to foods with greater or lesser amounts of salt. If you have hot cereals for breakfast, you will notice that a day or two of omitting the salt called for on the package is all it takes to get used to the lower-sodium taste. Likewise, try vegetables without added salt, and see how easy it is to modify this taste.

Taste Repetition

Taste repetition is important. Some years ago, on a trip to Mexico's Yucatan peninsula, the chef of a beach hotel proudly presented a plate of black beans with *salsa*. He was fond of the

savory beans and the carefully prepared sauce of fresh tomatoes, peppers, and onions. Obviously, this was a much healthier
meal than the steak and french fries that most American
tourists might eat. With my American palate geared to very
different kinds of foods, the subtle flavors of the black beans
and salsa escaped me. But after trying it again a few times, I
came to see why he was so proud of this age-old Mexican dish.
The chance to repeat tastes is the key to acquiring new tastes.

In trying low-fat foods and ethnic dishes, allow yourself
several chances to get used to new flavors. Some foods that
may seem strange or exotic the first time you taste them can
soon become favorites.

It takes time to get away from a "fat addiction." Don't be
surprised if you find yourself craving fat, dreaming of Crisco
mountains and lard-filled valleys, with islands of chicken fat
in rivers of grease. You may find yourself looking longingly
through the windows of McDonald's. Don't worry. This, too,
shall pass.

Watch for Hidden Fat

On the kitchen counters of America, cooks are carefully
trimming the fat off roasts. What they may not realize, however, is that farmers have been working long and hard to
"marble" fat throughout the beef, so that it is permeated by the
fatty taste. As long has you are eating meat—even lean meat—
you are getting far more fat than you would get from truly
healthful foods, such as vegetables, breads, pastas, beans, and
fruits. Even poultry and fish contain inherent fat. Fried foods
are packed with fat too. A 95-calorie potato made into french
fries emerges from the cooking vat with nearly 300 calories.

"Sauté" in Water

If you find yourself making sauces or casseroles by sautéing
onions, garlic, or other vegetables in oil, try using water
instead. Simply use a small amount of water in a saucepan,
and simmer onions, garlic, etc. for a few minutes. The taste is
lighter because it is oil-free.

Read the Label

Labels on food packages tell you how much fat is in a product and what kind of fat it is. First of all, a word about types of fat. It has long been known that certain types of fat—particularly animal fat—are worse than others when it comes to their tendency to promote heart disease. In addition, a few vegetable oils are high in saturated fats. These are the tropical oils (palm oil, palm kernel oil, and coconut oil) and hydrogenated oils. The main point, though, about fats and oils is this: reduce them all. All oils are high in calories, and all cause a variety of health problems.

When you read the list of ingredients on a package, the ingredient which is used in the largest amount is listed first. The ingredients used in smaller amounts are listed in descending order. So a jar of spaghetti sauce whose ingredients were listed as "water, tomato paste, onions, olive oil . . ." would probably contain less oil than a brand whose ingredients were listed as "water, olive oil, tomato paste, onions . . ."

How to Caculate Fat Content

When we choose to limit our fat intake to 10 percent or 20 percent or 30 percent of our diet, how do we figure what our fat intake is? I don't recommend bringing a calculator every time you go out for a snack, but you may wish to calculate the amount of fat in certain foods, and it's useful to check on foods you commonly eat.

Simply check the "calories from fat" listed on the nutritional label and divide by the total calories.

Exploring a New World of Foods

There is a whole world of healthful, delicious foods waiting for us, made principally from grains, legumes, and vegetables. Many of them are already familiar: spaghetti, chili, soups, and burritos. Some are exotic-sounding new foods. All are delightful. This is the time to explore the new world of eating choices.

Try out new foods. Don't simply read about them. Think in terms of action: try new recipes, try ethnic restaurants, and recruit friends or family members to join you in making a meal. The key is to think less about making resolutions and more about practical actions that can solidify changes. You can use America's favorite pastime—shopping—to help improve your menu.

As healthful eating becomes second nature, you will start to notice that you feel different physically and mentally. If you have been overweight, enjoy the feeling of slimming down. As blood pressure problems come under better control, medications are often reduced or eliminated by your doctor, and their side-effects will subside as well. As cholesterol levels drop, people with heart problems begin to feel younger. Your friends will notice how good you look, and that will make you feel better too.

Explore International Cuisine

Treating yourself to international restaurants is not only fun; but helps show that delicious foods can be healthful as well, and helps you adapt your tastes. Italian, Chinese, Japanese, Mexican, Indian, Thai, Ethiopian, Middle-Eastern, and many other exotic restaurants offer delicious foods. They will give you ideas for dishes you can make at home. Exploring these foods can help you develop new tastes.

At an Italian restaurant, have spaghetti with tomato sauce. It contains only about 350 calories and has no cholesterol and little fat. At a Mexican restaurant, have a bean burrito with Spanish rice. At a Chinese restaurant (including Szechuan or Hunan) look at the many exotic vegetable dishes. Try the different varieties of bean curd, in which tofu is transformed into deliciously spiced, savory meals. (Tell them not to add meat, or they very likely will, in anticipation of American tastes.) Indian restaurants feature an endless variety of elegant foods from soups to curries, rice dishes, and exotic breads. At Middle-Eastern restaurants, *hummus* makes a delicious sandwich or dip (see page 236 for recipe). Ethiopian restaurants have become very popular in Washington, D.C., and other large cities. They transform lentils, split peas, vegetables, and spices into a stunning and unique banquet served on a delicate soft bread. Japanese, Thai, Vietnamese, and other Asian countries have traditions of delicious foods combining rice with carefully prepared vegetables.

One tip at Asian restaurants: at the end of their menus, you will often find a vegetable section. These are not side-dishes. They are vegetable entrees and offer a variety of tasty meals.

Each tradition has its own favorite ingredients and flavorings. Learning to use them is a delightful way to expand your culinary repertoire. You will find cookbooks for each cuisine at the library and most large bookstores. Choose the best dishes and feel free to adapt them as needed.

One word of caution: Chefs are all too eager to please the American penchant for greasy foods by smearing butter, oil, chunks of meat, and globs of cheese on otherwise healthful foods. Health-conscious customers should let their needs be known.

As you experience new cuisines, you may find that your food preferences shift from an emphasis on fat and protein toward new tastes. Some people get "hooked" on Szechuan, Mexican, Indian, or Italian food. Perhaps you will too.

Explore the Bookstore

One of the other things you can feel free to consume in unlimited quantities is cookbooks. There are many excellent ones. As William Castelli, M.D., of the Framingham Heart Study, says, try vegetarian cookbooks, as many as you can, until you find ten to twelve recipes you enjoy. Many of the recipes are low in fat and cholesterol, and are usually free of the contamination problems common in meats. Browse at the library or bookstore, and try new recipes to add to your routine. Also check the cookbook selection at the health-food store. Often you will find unusual and interesting books.

Explore the Health Food Store

Health food stores often have a selection of interesting foods that are not available in regular groceries. You will probably not want to do all of your shopping at such specialty stores, since many healthful foods can be found at regular grocery stores. But health food, gourmet, and Asian grocery stores carry some wonderful products you will want to try.

First of all, what is a health food store? Unfortunately, some stores function only as outlets for vitamins, so look around a bit. Even small towns now have stores that carry the products that larger groceries omit. Look in particular for the products listed in Chapter 12.

Expect to buy a few duds. The point of experimenting is not to have every product or every meal turn out wonderfully. Rather, you just want to try as many new possibilities as you can. Some health food stores would be glad to take your life savings, but ultimately you will save a great deal of money, because grains, beans, vegetables, and fruits are far cheaper than meats, dairy products, and other unhealthful foods.

A New Look At the Old Store

At the supermarket, browse through the sections of healthful but easy-to-prepare foods. Look at the varieties of whole grain breads and hot cereals that are now available. Try the many variations of wild rice or brown rice. They can be found in boxed dinners that are easy to make, yet very delicious. Some prepared spaghetti sauces are very tasty and cholesterol-free. Read the labels and pick out those lowest in fat.

Pick up a can of black beans. You may wish to cook dried beans (which takes several hours), but canned beans are a convenient way to taste many varieties. While some people (particularly those headed for coronary bypasses) regard beans as second-class foods, black beans are especially savory. You can find them with Progresso products or other canned beans at most grocery stores. Black beans, like most other beans, are very low in fat and calories (not to mention low in cost) and contain no cholesterol, yet they are delicious topped with mild *salsa* which you will find in the Mexican foods section. Most stores stock a variety of brands of Mexican sauces ranging from mild to hot. Have beans with rice, whole grain breads, potatoes, or other starches.

You will find the produce section packed with foods that are free of cholesterol and low in fat, yet endlessly varied. Thanks to indoor growing, most seasonal vegetables are available year-round. Pick up some fresh basil to blend into a pesto sauce for pasta. Add broccoli, cauliflower, carrots, spinach, green beans, and other tasty vegetables to your daily routine. While you are at it, pick up some raisins, dates, bananas, strawberries, blueberries, peach slices, or cinnamon to top your hot cereal.

Vegetables are delicious and full of vitamins. At each lunch and dinner, try having at least two different vegetables, instead of one. Buy vegetables fresh or frozen. Some, such as fresh spinach and carrots, are delicious without cooking. When you do cook vegetables, steam or boil them in a small amount of water. Do not fry. Also avoid overcooking or adding butter, fat, margarine, or oil. Enjoy the unadulterated taste of freshly prepared vegetables, or, if you like, add a sprinkle of lemon or lime juice.

Check the endless varieties of exotic sauces, chutneys, mustards, and imported foods in the international and gourmet food sections.

To avoid making regrettable purchases, go to the grocery store after eating rather than before. Keep your shelves stocked with healthful foods. Certain items, such as canned beans, spaghetti, and rice, keep indefinitely. When we are rushed or impulsive or simply want something convenient, it helps if we have healthful foods handy. If snacking is a problem for you, store foods out of sight. Planning prevents many lapses. Write out your menus at the beginning of each week. Plan for seven days worth of meals, and buy what you need for the week. This will help you eliminate impulse shopping and help you stick to your resolve.

Phasing Out Unhealthful Foods

So far we have been discussing how to bring new foods into your menu. Before long, however, you will also want to get the old ones out. Is change easy for you, or do you need a bit of time to get used to new things? Some people choose a gradual approach. Others like—or perhaps need—to make changes more rapidly. There are different ways to go about changing your eating habits. It helps to choose a method that suits your own needs. Here are three approaches to getting rid of the old, unhealthful foods:

Transition Foods: In psychological theory, there is the concept of *transitional objects*. A transitional object is something tangible that helps ease the pain of a major change. For children, for example, a teddy bear helps in the transition to independence. As children venture away from their parents, their teddy bears help them carry a semi-companion with them until they feel more secure. There are what we might call transition foods, as well. These are foods that help us over the gap from meat and dairy products to more healthful foods. They simulate the taste and texture of the offending foods, while actually being made from much more healthful ingredients.

Larger grocery and health food stores carry many of these foods. Check in the gourmet and dietetic aisles. You will find soy hot dogs, mock chicken, non-meat ground "beef," meatless chili, and a variety of "burgers" made from soybeans or other plant foods. These and other transition foods are described in Chapter 12. There are even ice cream substitutes which taste absolutely terrific. It is intriguing to see the technologies that have been put to work to lure you away from unhealthful foods.

These products generally substitute vegetable protein for animal protein. Some contain more vegetable oil than is desirable over the long-term; hence the term "transition" foods. Transition foods provide a lot of help when you are leaving behind old favorites, confronting urges to compromise your resolve, or entertaining friends who are eating in particularly unhealthful ways.

The Five-Step Approach: This approach breaks the overall change into distinct stages. Each step is significant without being overwhelming. Allow a month or more to adapt to each step before going on to the next. But do not stay too long at any of the intermediate steps and expect to achieve maximal gains. The strongest gains come at the completion of all steps.

Step 1. Add grains and legumes to your dietary routine. This step adds foods that are rich in complex carbohydrates and fiber, low in fat, and free of cholesterol. Try whole grain breads, rice dishes, hot cereals, and savory bean or lentil dishes.

Step 2. Add more vegetables. Drop by the produce department of your grocery store. Like grains and legumes, they're high in complex carbohydrates and fiber with little or no fat and no cholesterol. Frozen vegetables are fine as well. Keep a generous variety on hand.

Step 3. Eliminate meat, chicken, and fish. In so doing, you will have cast out major sources of fat, cholesterol, and calories. If you are uncertain as to the need for this, review the chapters on heart disease, cancer, and common illnesses. Make the step a complete one. Little bits of chicken and fish tend to lead to more and more. Getting rid of these products entirely makes for an easier transition, and a more healthful diet overall. At this stage, you may wish to try some transition foods as well.

Step 4. Eliminate eggs and dairy products. Dairy products include milk, cream, cheese, sour cream, yogurt, whey, and casein (a milk protein, often used as sodium caseinate in commercial products). Most dairy products are loaded with fat and cholesterol. In addition, many people have subtle, or not so subtle, allergies to milk proteins, which are present even in low-fat products. Sniffles, postnasal drip, canker sores, and other problems are often due to milk allergies. If you think that milk products are necessary to avert osteoporosis, you are behind the times. See Chapter 6. Many people feel much better getting dairy products off the menu.

Step 5. Minimize vegetable oils. Instead of frying in oil, sauté foods in small amounts of water. Eliminate added oils from recipes. Avoid high-fat foods such as potato chips, french fries, and oily salad dressings.

The 21-Day Plan: This plan is for those who like to think short-term. You will make dramatic changes, but will do so for only three weeks. You will make maximum gains during that period and can then decide whether or not to continue for another three-week period.

Here is how to proceed: In planning meals, emphasize grains, legumes, vegetables, and fruits. At the same time, omit all meats, dairy products, fried foods, and vegetable oils. Chicken and fish are to be omitted as well in this plan. This sounds like a big change, and it is. You are getting rid of all the major sources of fat and cholesterol and adding the best foods for weight control and prevention of illness. Remember, we are only doing this for three weeks. You will show yourself what you can do.

This is the method John McDougall uses in helping his patients change their eating habits. He says, "I try to help people to understand that they have to give up the delicacies for a while until they get better. I put it to them that way. Instead of saying, 'For the rest of your life you're never going to eat another piece of turkey again,' I'll say, 'All you've got to do is do it for three weeks. I want you to be real strict and leave all those delicacies alone for three weeks, and then we'll talk about it.' They'd come back in three weeks. They'd be down 8-10 pounds, their cholesterol would be down, their blood pressure would be down, and so on. I'll say 'OK, you've done real well, let's go on, let's keep doing it.' And after a while they develop a taste for the new things, and the old things—they'd learn to live without them."

This is not a time to make halfway changes. For three weeks, be strict. You will want to give yourself the best chance for maximum improvements. Cheating only leads to more temptation. If you want to modify things and compromise, do so at the end, after you have given yourself three weeks on the optimal program. You will probably find that by not compromising you will reach your goal faster than you had imagined possible.

At the end of three weeks, see how you feel. If you like, go back and try the old foods again. You will probably notice that meats, dairy products, and fried foods have a distinctly greasy taste. On the other hand, if you like the way things are going, you do not need to stop. You can "re-enlist" for another three weeks. Then size up your gains. If you choose to continue, you will make more progress. If you decide to permanently revert back to unhealthful eating, your progress will be lost. By keeping the time periods to three weeks, there isn't the feeling that one's favorite indiscretions have to be lost forever.

Sticking to Your New Meal Plan

Check your progress. As you begin to change your diet, you may notice several things. You may feel better mentally, that is, your spirits may be a bit brighter than before. For reasons that have never been quite clear, people who eat well often report feeling more energetic, with more stable moods. Whether it is due to more stable blood sugars, reduced viscosity ("thickness") of the blood, or less constipation and other physical complaints, there can be a real sense of well-being.

You cannot feel blood pressure or cholesterol, but if you see your doctor after a few weeks of a new way of eating you may well find an improvement in both. You also cannot feel your cancer risk, but that has been improving since the day you first started working on your food preferences. If you were overweight, you will probably have begun a steady decline in your weight. But do not be overeager; a slow, steady decline is best for permanent weight control.

Get some social support. Ask your family or a friend to join you as you remodel your eating habits. Family and friends keep us afloat during periods of uncertainty. Bringing others along helps solidify the motivation for change, allows us to share information, and helps us persevere during periods of difficulty. They will reap tremendous benefits just as you will.

Social support is the key ingredient in the most challenging life-style change programs, from Alcoholics Anonymous to addiction clinics to smoking cessation programs. It is just as important in dietary change.

Keep things simple. It is easier to focus on one or two major changes in the diet than several minor ones.

A complicated list of ideas, such as "Eat less fat, less cholesterol, more fiber, more beta-carotene, more cruciferous vegetables, less protein, fewer contaminants, more vitamin C, etc., etc.," is very hard to remember. You can accomplish all these goals much more simply by keeping in mind the idea of choosing foods from plants rather than animal sources. I often tell my patients to think of a *low-fat vegetarian diet* as the ideal. In that simple phrase are summed up most of the principles you need.

Many people find it easier to make a clean break from unhealthful foods, rather than continuing to include them in small quantities. Just as it is difficult for many people to smoke occasional cigarettes without being hooked, a small amount of meat in the diet for some people leads to continued eating of larger amounts than intended.

Focus on your long-term gains. We plan for our children's college education while they are still in diapers. We save for our old age. We work toward our long-range goals through education, finance, and career plans. But all too often, we are on a short-sighted diet. We eat as if we were death row convicts savoring an endlessly gluttonous last meal. We eat in such a way that, just as our families are maturing and we are able to profit from the fruits of our labor, we become too ill to enjoy them. We become overweight and toy with cancer and heart attacks.

Eating right is an investment. It is important for us and also tremendously important for our families. The second best gift we can give our children is to change our own diets so that we can be alive and well as they grow through life. The best gift is to help them develop a taste for foods that will keep them healthy.

See foods for what they are. Use concrete images to help solidify your resolve. Think in graphic terms: grains, beans, vegetables, and fruits are clean and healthful sources of protein, carbohydrate, vitamins, and fiber. Meats, on the other hand, are muscle tissues taken from carcasses. They are loaded with calories, cholesterol, and fat, and are often infected with live bacteria.

Trouble-Shooting

In the last few sections, we have looked at principles for bringing in new foods and getting rid of dangerous old ones.

In this section, we will look at some of the trouble spots we can hit along the way and how to handle them.

Handling Cravings

Cravings have a biological purpose. They guide us to respond to important needs. If we lose our air supply, we crave oxygen. After a day or two without water, we crave water. Craving is the body's way of telling us that things are getting worse and it is time for desperate action. But the craving mechanism often kicks in at the wrong time, like a defective oil light on your car. The craving for, say, sweets or fatty foods tells us that things will get worse and worse if we do not satisfy its demand. But, in fact, things do not get worse. Unlike the desire for air or water, *food cravings generally do not escalate.* Eventually, they simply go away. So see cravings for what they are: false alarms that will turn off shortly.

Unfortunately, we tend to respond to all cravings as emergencies. Cravings may lead to impulsive binging. Binging, in turn, deflates our self-esteem. We feel as if we simply cannot control what we eat.

A few points should be kept in mind in handling cravings:

First of all, do not use food as your only source of "nourishment." The more fun we have in the rest of our lives, the less we use food as a solution for other problems.

Second, develop an eating routine. Skipping meals makes cravings all the more likely.

Third, when cravings occur, fill up on healthful foods. Have some bread, unbuttered popcorn, cereal, or other foods you feel comfortable with. Cravings tend to occur when you are most hungry. As hunger diminishes, cravings fade away as well.

Fourth, identify the type of craving you experienced. If you found yourself longing for sweets, add more complex carbohydrates to your meals. Brown rice, whole grain bread, and cereals can provide the carbohydrate your body craved in a more healthful form.

Don't let slips steer you off course. Everyone goofs once in a while. Forgive yourself, and return to your new way of eating. The real mistake is letting one slip become an excuse for a second or third indiscretion or for abandoning healthy eating altogether.

Be patient with yourself. It takes a long time to become unhealthy. It takes time to become healthy again. There is no reason to be discouraged if you do not change instantly. This is particularly true for weight loss. Weight loss is always gradual. Some might feel discouraged if they have not rapidly rid themselves of all the excess weight they have accumulated. But the key is to stay in the right direction. As long as one is improving, gradual improvement is just fine.

Dining Out

When dining out, the selection of restaurants is key. If your boss asks you to lunch or friends invite you out after work, suggest a restaurant where healthful foods are available. Italian, Chinese, Mexican, and other international restaurants are available in cities and towns of all sizes and usually have meatless meals. American restaurants often offer vegetable plates and salad bars.

If you do not see what you would like on the menu, ask the waiter. Requests for vegetable plates, vegetarian foods, and changes in menu items are common. All good restaurants are able to handle them, although the menu may not yet reflect the full range of their capabilities. Lots of restaurants have some spaghetti and tomato sauce on the shelf, just waiting to be asked for. While dining with my parents at a Chinese restaurant in Fargo, North Dakota, I asked for bean curd Szechuan style. The management had never been asked for this tofu dish by the largely Scandinavian clientele, but they often prepared it for themselves. They were pleased to be able to serve the authentic Chinese dish.

Travel

Hotels and airlines all too often cater to the most unhealthful eating habits. A recent report in the *Journal of the American Medical Association* analyzed airline meals and determined that airline food posed a statistically greater danger to the average passenger than the possibility of a crash! When you book your flight ask for a vegetarian meal. All major airlines have them, and they are far better than the regular meals.

When I travel, I always look for ethnic restaurants, which are available virtually anywhere, and I do not hesitate to ask for foods that are not on the menu. Chefs want to please their customers and are usually happy to modify the menu a bit. My suitcase often holds a dried soup mix or instant oatmeal which can be mixed with hot water, even in flight. Hotels almost always have oatmeal that can substitute for morning eggs and bacon.

For fast-food fans, there are several possibilities. Taco shops have bean burritos which are usually cholesterol-free if they hold the cheese. Pizza restaurants can make a pizza with all the vegetable toppings (green peppers, mushrooms, onions, olives, etc.), extra sauce and no cheese. Often they can also make spaghetti with tomato sauce, even if it does not appear on the menu. Burger franchises can make a "veggie burger" with all the fixings but without the meat patty. Sandwich shops can make a vegetarian sub.

When Friends Give You Trouble

There is no topic more likely to attract unsolicited advice than food. Friends and relatives will routinely want you to eat more of this or less of that. Bad advice is given at least as freely as helpful advice. Some patience with such advice is usually required. Be glad that these friends care about you. They are trying in their own inaccurate way to look out for your health.

Your family and friends may not join you instantly as you change your way of eating. It is hard to let go of habits. And like any other loss, acceptance comes in stages. You may know of Elisabeth Kubler-Ross and her work helping people to deal with death and bereavement.[2] She wrote that, at first, we reject what has happened. But eventually, we come to terms with the situation. We have much the same reactions to lesser threats and losses too, and they can be understood in much the same way. When friends give you trouble about your new way of eating, you may find it useful to think of stages of acceptance of any new set of circumstances, including a change in eating habits. Kubler-Ross identified five stages of acceptance:

Denial. People find all kinds of ways of avoiding the facts, including ridicule.

Anger. In the attempt to make the message go away, there will be occasional attempts to "attack the messenger."

Bargaining. If we have to change, we hope to do so as little as possible. But we begin to make a few concessions.

Depression. As half-hearted attempts at bargaining fail, the facts are more stark than ever and demand to be taken seriously.

Acceptance. Having ridiculed and denied and fought and bargained our way along, we have finally accepted the need to change.

Everyone is in the process of change. Far too many are still in the stage of denial. But the facts about foods and health are becoming more widely understood, and many people are now well along in the process of change. So if someone should make fun of your way of eating (or as happened to me, you ask for tofu at the grocery store and the clerk says *"Toad food?* You want *toad food?"*), just remember that ridicule is part of the first stage of acceptance.

At a Friend's House

You have been invited to a holiday party. You anticipate that the food will be full of fat and cholesterol, but you do not want to offend your host by gagging at the sight of cholesterol croquettes or lard fajitas.

Here is the way I deal with this challenge, and I have never found it to fail. At the time of the invitation or shortly thereafter, I say that I would love to come, but since I am a vegetarian and certainly did not want to put them to any trouble, I would like to bring something along or to help with the cooking. Invariably, they decline my offer of help and tell me "My son is a vegetarian," or "My husband is trying to lower his cholesterol," so the idea of more healthful eating is clearly not alien. Most people are very curious about nutrition. This is far better than surprising the hosts at the last minute or destroying your own principles and your health.

Defenses That Block Progress

Defenses are used all day, every day by each of us. Defenses are the psychological maneuvers we use automatically to keep ourselves from feeling anxiety. We defend ourselves against our own impulses and against threats from the outside world. Defenses are used to solve conflicts. For example, perhaps we want to eat a big, juicy steak. And we know that that kind of food will kill us sooner or later. What do we do?

Denial: We use denial: "I won't get a heart attack," we say. "I'm strong as an ox; that couldn't happen to me." Denial is a primitive, but common defense. When reality is too unpleasant, we simply block it out. Suddenly, fatty foods and cigarettes do not cause cancer, at least not for us. We are not headed for a heart attack, and we are not overweight, in spite of what the scale may show. Denial can coexist with a superficial awareness of danger. For example, a person may be well-aware of the dangers of smoking but continue to do so because denial blocks out the immediacy of the threat. Happily, denial can be eroded by learning more about the dangers at hand. The more we are confronted with the real dangers of unhealthful foods, the less we can pretend that they do not exist.

There are other defenses too. Go on a "seek and destroy" mission for these defenses. Look for them in your friends. You will find they are everywhere.

Rationalization: When there is no good reason to do what we are doing, we invent one. The human brain has the capacity for using logic even when it bears no relationship to reality. "A little bit won't matter," we say as we dig in to high-cholesterol, high-fat foods. "I'll change next week," "I can't live without ——," and "People have always eaten this way" are common rationalizations that, while patently untrue, alleviate our worries. Rationalizations cannot stand up to the facts. So make sure you are well-informed.

Suppression: This simply means forcing oneself not to think about a desire. For some it is an effective way of handling momentary food urges, although not so effective as understanding them and gratifying them appropriately, or preventing their occurrence with a sound and satisfying eating routine.

Humor: Humor is one of the more "healthful" defenses. With humor, we acknowledge reality. It can be used to diffuse an unacceptable urge, for example in laughing and talking about "forbidden foods" instead of actually eating them.

If we can identify the psychological maneuvers that maintain unhealthful habits, we have taken the first step toward setting them aside.

Ideas That Block Progress

A single mistaken notion can defeat a mountain of evidence. Here are the most common ideas that discourage more healthful eating habits.

1. Foods aren't that important; your health just depends on your heredity.

Only a small percentage of people have a genetic predisposition toward elevated cholesterol. Hereditary factors are probably of even less significance in cancer risk. A tendency to overweight is, to an extent, inherited, but significant changes in the diet can help control weight regardless of one's heredity.

2. I'm too old to change.

As far as your coronary arteries are concerned, you are never too old. Evidence suggests that even established atherosclerosis can be reversed by lowering your cholesterol level. Cancer risk can be reduced and your weight can drop too, even if you have been heavy for years.

3. I'll become anemic if I eat less meat.

That would be called an old wives' tale, except that it is often promoted by poorly informed doctors, most of whom are not actually old wives. Vegetables and grains are rich in iron. Blood cells form perfectly well with the protein and vitamins found in plant sources. Anemia is no more likely on a well-balanced vegetarian diet than on a meat diet. On the other hand, people who rely on dairy products for their nutrition may, in fact, become anemic. Dairy products are very low in iron.

Meat is an undesirable source of iron and protein. Not that it is not rich in both, but it inherently contains lots of cholesterol and fat, the last things you need in your iron or protein sources. Vitamin B-12 is an issue for people who consume no animal products at all. This is discussed in detail on Chapter 10.

4. Changing my diet would mean giving up the pleasures of life.

First, cholesterol-free foods can be a savory *addition to your life*. Many people have never tasted international delicacies and creative American cuisine until encouraged to do so for reasons of health.

Meats are not what people generally enjoy so much as the sauces, herbs, and spices we use on them. Meatless foods can likewise be deliciously prepared.

The pleasures of life are far greater when you enjoy them in a slim, healthy body. You can also enjoy them a good bit longer.

5. If you avoid meats, you have to carefully complement vegetable proteins in order to get enough.

Protein sources naturally add to each other when we eat. You need not do so consciously. If you were to eat literally only one thing day after day, such as corn, and absolutely nothing else, you would be at risk for a deficiency. Obviously, no one eats that way. Our meals tend to be mixtures. As long as you are eating a variety of foods and getting enough calories to maintain your weight, a protein deficiency is extremely unlikely.

The idea of carefully complementing proteins was promoted by Frances Moore Lappe in the first edition of *Diet For a Small Planet* (Ballantine, 1971). In a later edition, she corrected the mistake. Unfortunately, many people seem to remember the older edition. As shown in Chapter 6, people are healthier if they eat more modest amounts of protein than most Americans routinely consume.

6. I'll get weak if I don't eat meat.

Bulls, stallions, elephants, and gorillas are all vegetarians. Their tremendous strength develops without an ounce of meat or dairy products. But a person who eats large quantities of meat will be weak indeed if atherosclerosis leads to a stroke. And atherosclerosis is a major contributor to impotence.

The body does not differentiate animal proteins from vegetable proteins as far as building muscles is concerned. We can get more than enough protein from plants.

Chapter 12

Food Ideas and Recipes

In the long evolution of foods, each culture has worked out unique ways to prepare and season foods. By selecting from among the best of these, we can have foods that are both healthy and delicious.

Transition Foods

As we saw in the last chapter, transition foods help us make the switch from high-fat meat and dairy products to healthier foods. Some can become part of your permanent menu. Others contain more vegetable oil than is desirable over the long-term and are really only to be used in the transition toward healthy eating. Even so, they allow you to explore and try new kinds of foods. Health food stores and larger groceries carry many of these foods.

Meat Substitutes: Instead of ground beef in recipes, try textured vegetable protien. Textured vegetable protein is made from soy flour with the fat removed. It has a long shelf life and works very well in spaghetti sauces, chili, tacos, etc. (See the recipe for *Spaghetti Balls* on page 247).

Try frozen or canned vegetarian "hot dogs." A number of companies make tasty tempeh "burgers," a soybean product (see page 225). They should be heated or baked, rather than fried.

Seventh Day Adventist food stores carry hundreds of transition foods, ranging from non-meat hot dogs and burgers to simulated ham, chicken, and just about everything else. Worthington and Loma Linda products feature a number of meat substitutes, usually canned, and are found in the health or gourmet section of grocery stores.

Progresso makes an eggplant appetizer that tastes very much like barbecued beef and works very well on a sandwich.

Dairy Substitutes: There are also transitional foods for dairy products. If you are fond of ice cream, try Tofutti, Ice Bean, or the other delicious non-dairy, ice-cream-like treats, available at many groceries and health-food stores. Rice and soy milks have entered a new age. Westsoy, Edensoy, Rice Dream, and other brands are delicious, lower in fat than cow's milk, and free of cholesterol. These non-dairy milks come in a variety of flavors and go very well on cereal. If you drink coffee, try rice milk. And try the recipe for cholesterol-free *Tofu Sour Cream* on page 249.

Cheese substitutes: Nutritional yeast (saccharomyces cerevisiae) is a good source of protein and B vitamins. It is bright yellow, comes in powder or flakes, is easily digestible, and lends a cheesy flavor to recipes. Try the *"Cheese" Sauce* recipe on page 249 with macaroni or on top of a pizza.

In addition, more and more soy "cheeses" are found on the market. Many of them are delicious, but they are high in fat and not recommended for more than transitional use. Many of them also contain casein, the milk protein, so check the label.

Modifying Recipes

Oil: In recipes calling for added oil, this can often be reduced or eliminated. Instead of sautéing foods in oil, try sautéing in water. For example, many recipes call for sautéing garlic or onions in oil. Instead, try putting about ½ cup of water in a saucepan, and adding the garlic and onions. In 10-

15 minutes, they will be nicely cooked without the added calories of oils.

Salt: When recipes call for salt, reduce or eliminate the salt called for. In recipes that call for tomato sauce, substitute tomato paste or puree, which are much lower in salt.

Meat: Use textured vegetable protein for a cholesterol-free meat substitute that is a good replacement for ground beef in sauces, chili, etc. (see previous section on "Meat Substitutes"). In Mexican dishes, pinto beans substitute well for meat. In some recipes, such as lasagne, casseroles, spaghetti sauces, etc., the meat can simply be eliminated.

Egg Substitutes: In baked goods, use Egg Replacer, available at natural foods stores. Most egg substitutes available at grocery stores simply omit the yolk, which is were the egg's cholesterol is found, and retain the white. An egg-sized bit of tofu also substitutes well for eggs in baking.

New Foods to Get To Know

There is a wealth of new nutritious foods you can incorporate into your diet. Since some of them may be unfamiliar to you, the following list will help you get to know them a bit. Some are found at your regular grocery. Others are mainly found at health food stores.

Brown rice: Rice is extraordinarily nutritious. It is low in fat and rich in carbohydrate and fiber. But few people know how to make rice taste good. Often it comes out like styrofoam because the cook bought the wrong kind of rice and cooked it in the wrong way. Short-grain brown rice has a crisp nutty texture. Long-grain brown rice is a light accompaniment for summer dishes. See page 240 for a good basic recipe for cooking either type.

Hot cereals: If you thought that hot cereals came in only one or two varieties, just take a look. You will find all kinds to taste. Try the barley and rice varieties, in addition to the more usual oat and wheat cereals.

Packaged soy and rice milks: They come in a variety of flavors and taste terrific. Read the labels and choose the brands which are lowest in fat. You may wish to dilute them with water.

Breads: A variety of whole grain breads can be found. Try several kinds and see which you prefer.

Tofu: Also known as bean curd, tofu takes on any flavorings that are cooked with it. It lends itself to many uses, from main dishes and salad dressings to desserts. It's sold in rectangular blocks and comes in different textures, from firm to soft. Although it contains no cholesterol, traditional varieties of tofu have a rather high fat content, so they should be used as a transition food. There are some lower fat varieties now available.

Tempeh burgers: Tempeh is a traditional Indonesian food made from soy beans. Tempeh "burgers" are simply patties which have been marinated and spiced. They can be baked or heated in various ways, and can make a breakfast patty, a sandwich filling, or an ingredient in stews and many other dishes.

Pasta: Get to know pastas. Spaghetti, macaroni, rotini, ditalini, and a multitude of other forms of pasta make low fat, cholesterol-free, tasty feasts. Pasta's reputation for being high in calories is entirely undeserved. It is only the high-fat toppings that are too often used—butter, oils, ground beef, etc.—that are high in calories. Properly prepared, pastas are both healthy and delicious.

Wild Rice: Wild rice is delicious and rich in fiber, yet low in calories. Although not a true rice, it goes well with any dish. Many flavorful varieties are available, some with added seasonings and cooking instructions. Simply follow the package directions and enjoy.

Sauces: Try the innummerable sauces and flavorings available on the specialty shelves, from Asian soy sauces, to Indian chutneys, to Latin American salsas. Miso is a rich, salty paste made from soybeans. It is a fermented food, varying in color and taste from light and slightly sweet to dark and robust. The Japanese use a teaspoonful in a cup of hot water to make a simple broth. You can use it to make fat-free gravies or to flavor sauces.

Sea vegetables: Get acquainted with sea vegetables, such as wakame, arame, dulse, hijiki, kombu, and nori. They are a rich source of vitamins and valuable minerals.

Soups: Healthy soups are now available in dried or canned varieties. Look for miso soup, lentil soup, or other varieties of meatless soup.

Packaged foods: A growing number of manufacturers are making delicious packaged foods that require minimal preparation, everything from frozen vegetarian dinners and canned imitation "meats" to burger mixes, and prepared grain dishes. Healthy eating was never easier.

Beans: Set aside whatever ideas you had about these modest members of the legume family. Exploring these foods will be very, very rewarding. Beans come in innumerable varieties and are very low in fat, high in protein and fiber, and free of cholesterol.

Go to the store and buy five cans of black beans. Most grocery stores have canned black beans, such as Progresso or Goya brands. I suggest five cans because the first time or two you may say, "What's so good about black beans?" But somewhere around the third or fourth time you try them—a similar lag time seems to occur for many foods—you will make them a staple in your menu.

Simply open the can, and heat the beans in a saucepan. Top with salsa, a Mexican tomato sauce which comes in mild or spicy versions. If you have trouble with spicy foods, stick to the mild varieties. Or top beans with chopped onions, green peppers, and/or tomatoes. Serve with brown rice, baked potato, bread, or on toast. Add a green salad or vegetable, and you have an excellent meal. See page 235 for tips on cooking dried beans.

Vegetables: Make vegetables part of your routine, rather than waiting to make that "special vegetable dish." Select fresh or frozen vegetables. Dark green, orange, and yellow vegetables are rich in beta-carotene and vitamin C. Green leafy vegetables are also a good source of minerals such as calcium. Cruciferous vegetables, such as broccoli, Brussels sprouts, cabbage, and cauliflower, contain additional natural substances that help prevent cancer.

Recipes

The recipes here are only the beginning. You can also try international and vegetarian cookbooks for more ideas.

Many are my own, while some of the more exotic recipes come from Camilla Meek, a nutritionally wise and artistic food preparer. Others were contributed by some of the Book Publishing Company authors, good cooks all.

Breakfast

Hot Cereals: Oatmeal and cereals are traditional American breakfast foods now making a comeback. Check out the nearest gourmet or health food store for new ideas. Don't ruin a fragrant bowl of hot cereal by topping it with milk. It is delicious plain, or topped with fruit, cinnamon, sorghum, etc.

Breads and Toast: Whole grain breads make great toast. A little jelly, jam, or cinnamon may be added, but avoid butter and margarine, which are mostly fat. Try toasted English muffins, especially whole wheat ones. Some are flavored with raisins and cinnamon.

Cold Cereals: The best cold cereals are those that contain whole grains and little else. Check the labels and avoid those with sugar and/or hydrogenated oils. Some people enjoy fruit juice on cereal or you can use soy milk or one of the dairy substitutes mentioned in the section on transition foods.

Beans on toast may sound strange but is a favorite breakfast in Mexico and parts of England. For the Mexican version, try black beans on toast with a little salsa or chopped tomatoes on top.

Tempeh patties: Patties can be broiled or heated in the oven to make a tasty breakfast patty. I prefer tempeh "burgers" which are tempeh mixed with various seasonings and are quite delicious.

Dinner for breakfast: There is nothing wrong with having a reprise of last night's scrumptious dinner the following morning. Sometimes leftovers make an excellent breakfast and are great time savers.

Pancakes: While fried foods should generally be avoided, it is far better to fry pancakes than eggs or sausage. If using a prepared mix, don't add eggs or milk, just add water. Use a non-stick cooking surface and, if necessary, a small amount of spray-on vegetable oil. For a special treat, add blueberries or finely chopped apples to the mix.

Scrambled Tofu

Scrambled tofu can replace scrambled eggs, but in the transition stage only, as it is too high in fat. Some delicious mixes can be found at your health food store, such as those by Fantastic Foods.

Crumble into a bowl:
   1 lb. firm tofu

Mix in with a fork:
   2 Tbsp. low sodium soy sauce
   1 Tbsp. Dijon mustard
   3 Tbsp. nutritional yeast flakes (page 223)

Heat a skillet over medium high heat. Add:
   1 Tbsp. vegetable oil

When oil is hot, stir in the tofu and heat for a few minutes. Serve hot on whole wheat toast.

This makes 4 generous servings.

Eggless Omelets

Combine in a blender:
   2 cups unbleached flour
   ⅓ cup nutritional yeast flakes (page 223)
   ½ tsp. baking powder
   3 cups water
   1 Tbsp. oil

Whip up batter until smooth. It can rest for 30 minutes to overnight in the refrigerator. Heat a 9" skillet and when hot put a few drops of oil on the bottom. Rotate the pan to coat the bottom. Pour ¼ cup of batter into pan and immediately tilt and coat the pan so batter forms an even layer over the whole bottom. Cook over medium high heat until the top starts to dry up and edges loosen. Slide pancake turner under it, flip over, and cook the other side. Besides serving as little omelets, these can be rolled up like crepes. They are especially good wrapped around some sautéed mushrooms or ratatouille.

Soups

Delicious and nourishing for lunches, before meals, or between meals.

Prepared Soups: A number of high-quality, commercially prepared soups are available. Hain Naturals lentil soup is low in fat and low in sodium. Progresso Lentil Soup is likewise low-fat, although higher in sodium. Ramen noodle soups, once available only from Asian groceries, are now widely popular.

At the health food store you'll find some delightful instant soups, such as Golden Couscous soups made by Nile Spice Foods, and Fantastic Noodle soups made by Fantastic Foods. Miso Cup soups are tasty instant miso soups.

Miso Soup with Wakame

Soak for a few minutes, then cut into strips:
   3" piece of wakame

Bring to a boil:
   4 cups water

To the water add the strips of wakame and:
   1 cup onions, diced

Simmer for 15 minutes.

Put a small amount of this broth into a cup and stir in:
   1½ Tbsp. miso

Add this to the soup and simmer a few minutes, but do not bring to a full boil. Put into bowls and sprinkle on 1 Tbsp. each of chopped scallions and parsley. You may wish to add chopped carrots or celery to the soup or serve it over small cubes of tofu.

Gazpacho

Cut into chunks:
3 ripe tomatoes
1 medium onion
1 cucumber
½ green pepper

Then add:
1 clove garlic, minced
1 cup tomato juice
2 Tbsp. lemon juice
4 ice cubes

Add salt and pepper to taste, and a dash of cayenne. The ice helps chill the soup which should be served cold.

Black Bean Soup

This is a thick, hearty soup that can be a meal in itself, with a chunk of bread and a tossed green salad as accompaniments.

Wash, sort and soak overnight:
1 lb. black or turtle beans

Drain the beans, place in a soup pot with:
3 quarts fresh water
1 bay leaf

Bring the beans to a boil over high heat, then reduce heat to low. Cook 1½ to 2 hours or until beans are tender.

In a saucepan steam:
½ cup water
1 large onion, chopped
5 cloves garlic, chopped
1 green pepper, chopped

When the vegetables are soft, add to the soup with:
2 tsp. cumin
2 tsp. oregano
1 tsp. salt
2 Tbsp. cider vinegar

Simmer together 30 minutes, covered. Place a scoop of cooked brown rice in each soup bowl, ladle in the soup. Pass a dish of chopped red onions to be sprinkled on top of each bowl.

Salads

You can be adventurous with new salads as these recipes incorporate grains, legumes, or even seaweed into delightful dishes.

Cucumber Arame Salad

(from Camilla Meek)

This is a delicious light salad seasoned with arame and a delightful dressing. Arame is a brown sea vegetable with a delicate flavor.

Peel and halve lengthwise:
   1 cucumber

Scoop out the seeds and slice into thin crescents. Spread slices out and sprinkle with salt. Transfer to a bowl and let stand 15 minutes. Drain thoroughly.

Meanwhile, soak for 10 to 15 minutes, until soft:
   1 cup arame
   1 cup water

Drain any excess water from arame, then combine with cucumber and a dressing made by mixing:
   2 Tbsp. lemon juice
   1 Tbsp. brown rice vinegar
   1 tsp. low sodium soy sauce
   2 Tbsp. water

You can substitute wakame for the arame; soak it and cut into strips.

Serves 4 to 6

Tabouli (Bulgur Wheat)

(from Judy Brown)

Let soak for 30 minutes or until water is absorbed:
1 cup boiling water
1 cup bulgur

Stir in:
1 cucumber, chopped
1 tomato, chopped
2 cloves garlic, minced
4 green onions, chopped
1 red pepper, chopped
½ cup parsley, minced

Mix for a dressing:
2 Tbsp. olive oil
juice of 1 lemon
handful of chopped fresh basil or mint

Toss well and chill.

Makes 6 servings

Ethiopian Tomato Salad

Combine in a bowl:
½ jalapeño pepper, seeded and minced*
¼ cup red onions, chopped
1½ Tbsp. lemon juice
¼ tsp. black pepper

Stir in:
3 ripe tomatoes, chopped

Add a little salt to taste. Chill and serve cold.

Serves 4 to 6

*Use gloves to handle hot peppers, to avoid skin irritation.

Tofu Salad

For a transition salad, we recommend you try tofu salad. It tastes very much like egg salad and makes a good sandwich filling. Try it in pita pockets with leaf lettuce.

Grate on the coarse side of a grater, or crumble into a bowl:
   1 lb. firm tofu

Add:
   1 stalk celery, finely chopped
   2 green onions, finely chopped

Stir in a little Nayonaise mayonnaise substitute to moisten, and:
   ¼ tsp. tumeric

Add salt to taste and a dash of pepper. Serve on lettuce or as a sandwich filling.

Makes 3 cups.

Beans

Cooking Dried Beans

Wash and sort the beans, removing any tiny stones or shrivelled beans. Soak beans overnight to soften them. Drain, add two to three times as much water as beans, and cook about two hours until tender. Add more water if needed. Black beans may take as much as six hours to be soft. If beans are not cooked long enough, they will be tough and flavorless.

A pressure cooker will reduce cooking time. Use 3 cups of water for each cup of soaked, dried beans. Black beans, pintos, and garbanzos should cook in 40 to 45 minutes. Split peas and lentils are best cooked without pressure.

Black Beans with Rice

Simmer for 10 minutes:
¼ cup onion, diced
1 cup tomatoes (fresh or canned), diced
½ cup green or red peppers, diced
½ cup mild canned chili peppers, diced
½ clove garlic, crushed

Add and simmer for at least 15 minutes:
4 cups cooked black beans

Add enough water to keep the beans from sticking.

Serve with a generous portion of steamed brown rice, adding Salsa Mexicana or any mild salsa over the top. Garnish with parsley and chopped tomatoes.

Salsa Mexicana

*Cilantro, a traditional condiment, adds an attractive and
zesty touch to any bean dish.*

Mix:
**1 tomato, diced
½ onion, diced
1 Tbsp. fresh cilantro, chopped
¼ cup chili peppers, diced**

Cilantro (the leaves of the coriander plant) is not always available in
your produce department and can be omitted. Or substitute chopped
parsley which looks very much like it, but adds a very different flavor.

Hummus

*A Middle Eastern pâté made from chick-peas (garbanzo beans), this is
an excellent sandwich filling, especially in pita bread. Or use it as a dip
for raw vegetables.*

Soak overnight:
1½ cups chick-peas

Rinse, add 4 cups water and cook about 1½ hours until tender, or use
3 cups canned chick-peas.

Mash together or combine in a processor:
**3 cups cooked chick-peas
1 clove garlic, minced
¼ cup tahini (ground sesame seeds)
juice of 2 lemons
dash of tamari or soy sauce
¼ cup fresh parsley, minced
¼ cup scallions, chopped
½ cup water
¼ tsp. black pepper or more, to taste
¼ tsp. salt or to taste**

Add a little more water, if needed, to get a smooth consistency. Serve
in pita pockets or on regular bread with chopped tomatoes, lettuce, or
sprouts.

Armenian Beans with Dill

(from Dorothy Bates)

Soak in several cups of water for 3 hours or overnight:
1 cup dried white lima beans

Drain, add 3 cups of fresh water, and boil 1 to 1½ hours until beans are tender.

In a saucepan, add:
½ cup water
3 cloves garlic, minced
1 stalk celery, thinly sliced
1 carrot, thinly sliced

Cook vegetables about 5 minutes until just tender. Toss with the drained beans and:
1 tsp. dill weed
1 tsp. salt or to taste

Pinto Bean Burritos

Pinto beans are available in cans or can be soaked and cooked. If a pressure cooker is not used, cooking time will be about 2 hours. Whole wheat or corn meal tortillas can be found in the dairy section of most markets.

Simmer in a sauce pan for 10 minutes:
1 onion, minced
½ green pepper, minced
2 cloves garlic, minced
1 tsp. cumin
¼ cup water

Meanwhile, drain 4 cups cooked pinto beans.

Heat the beans, then mash them, and add to the pan with:
1 tomato, diced
1 tsp. salt
¼ tsp. pepper

Stir and simmer for 15 minutes. Warm 8 large tortillas by lightly toasting on a dry, hot griddle for less than a minute each, or wrapping in a dish towel and heating in a strainer basket over boiling water for a few minutes. Place bean filling on tortillas, top with salsa, hot sauce, nutritional yeast, or shredded lettuce and roll up.

Indian Split Pea Dal

Simmer for 30 minutes or until tender:
1½ cups yellow split peas
3 cups water

Add more water if needed. In another saucepan, simmer for 15 minutes:
1 large onion, chopped
1 small green pepper, chopped
1 tsp. tumeric
½ tsp. curry powder
1½ tsp. black mustard seeds
½ cup water

Mix with the peas when tender, adding:
juice of 1 lemon
salt to taste

Serve over generous portions of brown rice. Chutney is a nice accompaniment.

Super Chili

Combine in a large saucepan or Dutch oven:
2-16 oz. cans whole tomatoes, crushed
3 oz. can tomato paste
1 large onion, chopped
1 green pepper, chopped
1 cup textured vegetable protein (See page 224)
    mixed with 1 cup boiling water
1 jalapeño pepper, minced
2 Tbsp. or more chili powder
1 to 2 tsp. cumin powder
2 tsp. garlic powder
1 tsp. oregano
¼ tsp. allspice

Cover pan and simmer for an hour. Taste and add salt if needed.
Add:
1 cup red kidney beans

Simmer 30 minutes to an hour more. This is even better reheated the next day. Serve on hot rice or, for an interesting switch, on top of spaghetti.

Lentil Burgers

This is a great substitute for meat burgers.
It contains no cholesterol and little fat.

Bring to a boil in a saucepan:
3 cups water
1 cup dried lentils
½ cup brown rice

Simmer for forty minutes, adding water if necessary.

Then mix in:
½ onion, chopped
2 cloves garlic, crushed
1 Tbsp. soy sauce

Form into patties and fry on a non-stick surface till browned on each side. Serve on a bun like a hamburger, with pickle, catsup, mustard, etc. The mix will keep about three days if refrigerated.

Grains

In most of the world, grains are a mainstay of the diet. Most widely used are rice, wheat, corn, barley, and buckwheat, and most are used in an unrefined state. Once you start using brown rice and other whole grains, you'll find they have more texture and flavor than the polished white rice and white flour you were used to. Whole grains are complex carbohydrates, rich in nutrients, fiber, and protein and low in fat.

Brown Rice

This method of cooking lends a crisp, nutty texture to the rice.

Wash in a saucepan of cool water, then drain thoroughly:

1 cup short grain brown rice

Put pan on medium heat, and stir constantly until the rice dries, about one minute.

Add:

3 cups water

Bring to a boil, cover, and simmer about 40 minutes, until the rice is soft but retains a hint of crunchiness. Do not overcook. If any water remains, drain it off. Rice makes a delicious meal topped with beans, stir fried vegetables, or a curry. Or add flavor to rice with a few dashes of a low sodium soy sauce.

Pilaf, Greek Style

(from Dorothy Bates)

Rinse and drain:

1 cup short grain brown rice

Place saucepan over medium heat and stir rice until dry. Add to hot pan:

1 Tbsp. olive oil
½ cup onion, finely chopped

Cook a few minutes until the onion softens, then add:

3 cups hot vegetable stock*

Cover the pan, reduce heat to low, and simmer until the rice has absorbed the liquid, about 40 minutes.

Makes 4 generous servings

*Health food stores carry cubes or granules of dried vegetable stock. "Morga" is an excellent brand.

Spanish Rice

Cook 2 cups brown rice according to directions on page 240.

While it cooks, combine in a saucepan:

½ onion, chopped
½ green pepper, chopped
½ red bell pepper, chopped
3 cloves garlic, crushed
1 Tbsp. paprika
1 cup water

Bring to a boil and simmer 15 minutes. Mix well with:

6 oz. tomato paste
the cooked rice

Taste and add salt as needed.

Makes 8 servings.

Chinese Fried Rice

(from Dorothy Bates)

Have ready:
4 cups cooked brown rice

In a saucepan combine:
1 large onion, cut in thin half-moons
2 carrots, cut in thin, short sticks
2 stalks celery, thinly sliced on the diagonal
½ cup vegetable stock (see *Pilaf, Greek Style*, page 241)

Bring to a boil, cook 3 minutes, remove from heat. Vegetables will be crisp and just tender. Strain the vegetables, save the stock to add to soup or gravy.

Heat a large skillet or wok and when pan is hot add:
1 Tbsp. sesame oil
the precooked vegetables

Cook and stir a few minutes over medium high heat, then crumble in the cooked rice, mixing well.

Add:
2 to 4 Tbsp. low sodium soy sauce

If desired, add:
1 can sliced water chestnuts, drained

Garnish with:
4 green onions, chopped

Serve hot.

Makes 6 to 8 servings

Sweet and Sour Vegetables with Almonds

*You can make this flavorful sauce
while you are cooking 2 cups (raw) brown rice.*

Bake at 300° for 15 minutes:
   ½ cup almonds

Bring ½ cup water to a boil, add, and simmer for 5 minutes:
   1 onion, sliced into half moons
   1 green pepper, cut in 1" triangles
   1 tomato, chopped

Drain vegetables.

In a 2-quart saucepan, bring to a boil and boil for 2 minutes:
   ½ cup maple syrup
   ½ cup cider vinegar
   ½ cup catsup
   ¼ cup low sodium soy sauce

Add to sauce:
   1 Tbsp. cornstarch dissolved in ½ cup water

Cook a few minutes as it thickens. Add the vegetables and:
   1 cup unsweetened pineapple wedges

Add the almonds, cook a few minutes, and serve over generous helpings of the cooked brown rice.

Couscous

(from Dorothy Bates)

This golden grain is a staple of the Middle East. It is made from cracked semolina wheat and is good hot or served cold as a salad.

Bring to a boil:
3 cups water

Stir in:
2 cups couscous

Cover and remove from heat. Let stand 5 minutes, then fluff with a fork.

Bring to a boil:
½ cup water

Add:
1 carrot, thinly sliced, slices cut in half
1 sweet red pepper, chopped
¼ cup currants or golden raisins
¼ cup red onions, chopped

Cook three minutes so they are just tender.

Drain the vegetables and add to the liquid:
3 Tbsp. olive oil
juice of 1 lemon
2 tsp. maple syrup
1 tsp. Dijon mustard

Mix the couscous with the vegetables and sauce and serve warm. Leftovers make a great cold salad the next day.

Stir Fry Vegetables with Rice

Have an assortment of colorful vegetables ready. Parboil harder vegetables, such as carrots, green beans, broccoli, or cauliflower for just a few minutes. Save the liquid you parboil in to make the sauce. The vegetables should be just tender when served.

Have ready:
   1 onion, thinly sliced in half moons
   1 stalk celery, thinly sliced on the diagonal
   1 green pepper, thinly sliced
   1 carrot, cut in matchsticks
   1 cup broccoli florets*
   1 cup cauliflower florets

Bring 1 cup water to a boil, add carrots, broccoli, and cauliflower. Cover and boil just 3 minutes. Drain, pouring cooking liquid into a bowl.

Add to hot liquid:
   1 tsp. vegetable broth granules
   2 Tbsp. low-sodium soy sauce
   1 tsp. sorghum or maple syrup

Heat a wok or large skillet over medium high heat. When pan is hot, add 1 Tbsp. sesame oil, then quickly stir fry the onion, celery, and pepper for 2-3 minutes. Add the drained vegetables and stir fry a minute more. (If you like softer vegetables, put a lid on the pan and cook 1 or 2 minutes.) Stir in the sauce and let it bubble up, then remove pan from heat. Serve vegetables over plates of brown rice.

Stems of broccoli can be peeled, sliced and steamed for a tasty vegetable.

Spaghetti with Tomato Sauce

Combine in a kettle:
1 green pepper, diced
1 onion, diced
½ cup water

Simmer for 10 minutes.

Add:
1-16 oz. can plum tomatoes, chopped
2 small cans tomato paste
2 cups vegetable broth
2 cloves garlic, crushed
½ cup parsley, chopped
1 bay leaf
2 tsp. oregano
1 tsp. basil
½ tsp. salt
¼ tsp. pepper

Simmer, covered, for about 1 hour. For a thicker sauce, simmer uncovered another 30 minutes. If desired, add 8 oz. mushrooms, rinsed, cut in quarters.

Commercial Spaghetti Sauces: For those who do not have an hour to simmer a sauce, stores carry a variety. Read the labels and choose a brand that has no meat or cheese and is lower in fat and sodium.

Spaghetti Balls (or Burgers)

Here is a low-fat, no-cholesterol version of an old favorite.

Pour 1¾ cup boiling water over 2 cups dry textured vegetable protein and soak for 10 minutes.

Steam together for a few minutes:
½ cup water
1 small onion, diced

Mix onion with textured vegetable protein and stir in:
½ cup unbleached flour
1 tsp. salt
1 Tbsp. low-sodium soy sauce
½ tsp. chili powder
½ tsp. garlic powder
½ tsp. oregano

Shape this mixture into balls 1" in diameter, pressing firmly. Spray vegetable oil into a non-stick pan and cook balls until browned. Or shape into patties, fry lightly until brown, and serve in buns.

Makes 36 balls

Pasta al Pesto
(Pasta with Pesto Sauce)

(from Camilla Meek)

This pasta in delicate fresh basil sauce is one of my favorite meals. It takes less than 30 minutes to make and is always a big hit.

While bringing water to a boil for the pasta, you can make the sauce.

Place in a blender or processor:
1 bunch (1½ cups loosely packed) fresh basil
½ Tbsp. olive oil
1 clove garlic, minced
1 Tbsp. barley miso
2 Tbsp. walnuts or pine nuts
¼ cup water

Blend until a creamy consistency is reached, then add 2 more Tbsp. walnuts or pine nuts and mix just a second or two. Cook 1 pound spaghetti or linguini according to package directions and drain. Serve about 3 Tbsp. of sauce over each serving of pasta.

Pasta e Fagioli
(Pasta and Beans)

Soak in water to cover for at least 6 hours:
1 cup dried Great Northern beans

Drain, bring to a boil with 3 cups water and a bay leaf. Cook 1 to 1½ hours until tender, adding more water if needed.

Add:
6 cloves garlic, crushed
6 oz. tomato paste
½ tsp. rosemary or basil
1 cup water

Cook 30 minutes; it should be the consistency of thick soup. Taste and add salt as needed. Cook 1 pound of macaroni, ditalini, or broken spaghetti according to package directions. Put drained pasta into large soup bowls, then ladle the bean soup mixture over the pasta. There should be more pasta than beans.

Sauces

"Cheese" Sauce

See information on nutritional yeast, page 223.

Mix in a 2-quart saucepan:
½ cup nutritional yeast flakes
½ cup unbleached flour
1 tsp. salt
½ tsp. garlic powder

When dry ingredients are mixed, whisk in:
2 cups water

Cook over medium heat, whisking, until it thickens and bubbles. Cook 30 seconds more, then remove from heat and whisk in:
¼ cup oil
1 tsp. wet mustard

Sauce will thicken as it cools but will thin when heated. Good for a macaroni and cheese casserole, as a topping for lasagne, or a pan of enchiladas.

Tofu Sour Cream

A friend of mine participated in Dr. John McDougall's fitness program in Northern California and came back with this extraordinary recipe.

Blend in a food processor or blender until very smooth:
1 lb. tofu
juice of 1½ lemons
1 Tbsp. dill
1 tsp. salt

Keep chilled. Use it as a basis for an herb or spicy dip, or on burritos or baked potatoes. Try different brands of tofu, as the softer varieties work better.

Snacks
and
Beverages

Rounding out our a plan for healthy eating, remember that between-meal snacks and drinks can either be wise or unhealthy choices. For healthy snacks, try the following:

Popcorn: Although it has a reputation as "junk food," as long as oil and salt are not added, it is a healthy mix of carbohydrate, protein, and fiber. It is best prepared by a hot-air popper. Try it sprinkled with nutritional yeast.

Fruits: Grapefruits, apples, oranges, bananas, pears, peaches, strawberries—the list is endless. Enjoy the whole fruit, rather than just the juice, which concentrates the fruit sugars and omits the fiber.

Raw vegetables: A crunchy snack that takes little time to prepare. Besides the usual carrot and celery sticks, try sticks of cucumber and zucchini.

If your hunger recurs at the same time everyday, it may be that your meal schedule needs to be moved up a bit.

For beverages, water and tea are excellent choices. If you like, squeeze a little lemon or lime juice into a glass of water. Juices and soft drinks are permissible in limited quantities. Avoid diet drinks. Aspartame (NutraSweet®) is implicated in convulsions and raises the possibility of abnormal brain development in children. Pregnant women and children should steer clear. Adults should avoid it too. Replacing sugar with aspartame is like replacing margarine with motor oil.

Perrier, Evian, and other bottled waters are delicious and free of calories. Club soda is another popular no-calorie drink.

References

CHAPTER 1

1. Castelli WP. Epidemiology of Coronary Heart Disease, *Am J Medicine* 1984:76(2A):4-12.
2. Lipid Research Clinics Program. The Lipid Research Clinics Coronary Primary Prevention Trial Results, II. *JAMA* 1984:251(3):365-74
3. Pennington JAT, Church HN. 1989. *Food Values of Portions Commonly Used*. New York: Harper and Row.
4. National Research Council. 1982. *Diet, Nutrition and Cancer*. Washington, D.C.: National Academy Press.
5. Kinosian BP, Eisenberg JM. Cutting into cholesterol: cost-effective alternatives for treating hypercholesterolemia. *JAMA* 1988; 259(15):2249-54.
6. Grimm RH et al. Effects of thiazide diuretics on plasma lipids and lipoproteins in mildly hypertensive patients. *Annals of Internal Medicine* 1981; 94:7-11.
7. Johnson BF. The effects of thiazide diuretics upon plasma lipoproteins. *J Hypertension* 1986;4:235-9.
8. Fries ED, Materson BJ. Short-term versus long-term changes in serum cholesterol with thiazide diuretics alone. *Lancet* June 23, 1984; 1414-15.
9. von Schacky C, Fischer S, Weber PC. Long-term effect of dietary marine omega-3 fatty acids upon plasma and cellular lipids, platelet function, and eicosanoid formation in humans. *J Clin Invest* 1985; 76:1626-31.
10. Endres S, Ghorbani R, Kelley VE, et al. The effect of dietary supplementation with n-3 polyunsaturated fatty acids on the synthesis of interleukin-1 and tumor necrosis factor by mononuclear cells. *N Engl J Med* 1989; 320:265-71.
11. Beilin LJ. Vegetarian diet and blood pressure levels: incidental or causal association. *AM J Clin Nutr* 1988; 48: 806-10.
12. Ernst E, Pietsch L, Matrai A, Eisenberg J. Blood rheology in vegetarians. *Br J Nutr* 1986; 56:555-60.
13. Conn JW, Rovner DR, Cohen EL. Licorice-induced pseudoal-dosteronism: hypertension, hypokalemia, aldosteronopenia, and suppressed plasma renin activity. *JAMA* 1968:205:492-6.
14. Sacks FM, et al. Plasma lipoprotein levels in vegetarians. *JAMA* 1985; 254(10):1337-41.

CHAPTER 2

1 Lawrie GM, DeBakey ME. Coronary artery surgery study. *Circulation* 1983; 68:939-950 and 951-960.
2. DeBakey ME. The Coronary artery surgery study. *JAMA* 1984;252(18):2609-11.

CHAPTER 3

1 Moertel CG. On Lymphokines, Cytokines, and Breakthroughs. *JAMA* 1986;256:3141.
2. National Research Council. 1982. *Diet, Nutrition, and Cancer*. Washington: National Academy Press.
3. Armstrong B, Doll R. Environmental factors and cancer incidence and mortality in different countries, with special reference to dietary practices. *Int J Cancer* 1975;15:617-31.

4. Hirayama T. Epidemiology of breast cancer with special reference to the role of diet. *Prev Med* 1978; 7:173-195.
5. Rose DP, et al. Effect of a low-fat diet on hormone levels in women with cystic breast disease. 1. Serum steroids and gonadotropins. *JNCI* 1987;78(4):6233-26.
6. Ingram DM, et al. Effect of low-fat diet on female sex hormone levels. *JNCI* 1987;79(6):1225-29.
7. Kagawa Y. Impact of Westernization on the nutrition of Japanese: changes in physique, cancer, longevity and centenarians. *Prev Med* 1978;7:205-17.
8. Toniolo P, et al. Calorie-providing nutrients and risk of breast cancer. *JNCI* 1989;81:278-86.
9. Cramer DW, et al. Galactose consumption and metabolism in relation to the risk of ovarian cancer. *Lancet* 1989; 2:66-71.
10. Cramer DW, Xu H, Sahi T. Adult hypolactasia, milk consumption, and age-specific fertility. *Am J Epidemiol* 1994; 139:282-9.

CHAPTER 4

1. Pennington JAT. Bowes and Church's *Food Values of Portions Commonly Used*. New York, Harper and Row, 1989.
2. Suter PM, Schutz Y, Jequier E. The effect of ethanol on fat storage in healthy subjects. *New Engl J Med* 1992; 326:983-7.
3. de Castro JM, Orozco S. Moderate alcohol intake and spontaneous eating patterns of humans: evidence of unregulated supplementation. *Am J Clin Nutr* 1990; 52:246-53.
4. Danforth E, Jr., Sims EAH, Horton ES, Goldman RF. Correlation of serum triiodothyronine concentrations (T3) with dietary composition, gain in weight and thermogenesis in man. *Diabetes* 1975; 24:406.
5. Spaulding SW, Chopra IJ, Sherwin RS, Lyall SS. Effect of caloric restriction and dietary composition on serum T3 and reverse T3 in man. *J Clin Endocrinol Metab* 1976;42:197-200.
6. Mathieson RA, Walberg JL, Gwazdauskas FC, Hinkle DE, Gregg JM. The effect of varying carbohydrate content of a very-low-caloric diet on resting metabolic rate and thyroid hormones. Metabolism 1986; 35:394-8.
7. Welle S, Lilavivathana U, Campbell RG. Increased plasma norepinephrine concentrations and metabolic rates following glucose ingestion in man. Metabolism 1980; 29:806-9.
8. Deriaz O, Theriault G, Lavallee N. Fournier G, Nadeau A, Bouchard C. Human resting energy expenditure in relation to dietary potassium. *Am J Clin Nutr* 1991;54:628-34.
9. Foster GD, et al. Controlled trial of the metabolic effects of a very-low-calorie diet: short- and long-term effects. *AM J Clin Nutr* 1990; 51:167-72.
10. Stunkard AJ, Harris JR, Pedersen NL, McClearn GE. The body mass index of twins who have been reared apart. *N Engl J Med* 1990; 322:1483-7.

CHAPTER 5

1. Holmberg SD, Osterholm MT, Senger KA, Cohen ML. Drug-resistant Salmonella from animals fed antimicrobials. *New Engl J of Med* 1984; 311:617-22.
2. Holmberg SD, Wells JG, Cohen ML. Animal-to-man transmission of antimicrobial-resistant Salmonella: Investigations of U.S. outbreaks, 1971-1983. *Science* 1984;225:833-5.
3. Spika JS, et al. Chloramphenicol-resistant Salmonella newport traced through hamburger to dairy farms. *New Engl J Med* 1987;565-70.
4. St. Louis ME, et al. The Emergence of grade A Eggs as a major source of Salmonella enteritidis infections. *JAMA* 1988; 259(14):2103-7.

5. National Research Council. 1987. *Poultry inspection: the basis for a risk-assessment approach.* Washington, D.C.:National Academy Press.
6. Wempe JM, et al. Prevalence of Campylobacter jejuni in two California chicken processing plants. *Appl Environ Microbiol* 1983; 45:355-359.
7. Kinde H, et al. Prevalence of Campylobacter jejuni in chicken wings. *Appl Environ Microbiol* 1983; 45:1116-1118.
8. Cover TL, Aber RC. Yersinia entrocolitica. *New Engl J Med* 1989;321(1):16-24.
9. U.S. Department of Agriculture Food Safety and Inspection Service. *Nationwide beef microbiological baseline data collection program: steers and heifers,* October 1992-September 1993. Washinton, D.C.: U.S. Department of Agriculture, 1994.
10. U.S. Department of Health and Human Services. Concern continues about Vibrio vulnificus, *FDA Drug Bulletin* April, 1988; 18(1):3.
11. National Resources Defense Council. 1987. *Regulating pesticides in food: the Delaney paradox.* Washington, D.C.: National Academy Press.
12. National Resources Defense Council. 1989. *Intolerable Milk: pesticides in our children's food.* Washington, D.C.: National Resources Defense Council.
13. Hergenrather J, et al. Pollutants in breast milk of vegetarians. *New Eng J Med* 1981;304:792.
14. Baker RC, et al. Survival of Salmonella typhimurium and Staphylococcus aureus in eggs cooked by different methods. *Poultry Sci* 1983;62:1211-16.

CHAPTER 6

1. Brand JC, et al. Plasma glucose and insulin responses to traditional Pima Indian meals. *Am J Clin Nutr* 1990;51:416-20.
2. Barnard RJ, et al. Response of non-insulin-dependent diabetic patients to an intensive program of diet and exercise. *Diabetes Care* 1982;5(4):370-74.
3. Barnard RJ, et al. Long-term use of a high-complex-carbohydrate, high-fiber, low-fat diet and exercise in the treatment of NIDDM patients. *Diabetes Care* 1983;6(3):268-73.
4. Scott FW. Cow milk and insulin-dependent diabetes mellitus: is there a relationship? *Am J Clin Nutr* 1990:51:489-91.
5. Karjalainen J, Martin JM, Knip M, et al. A bovine albumin peptide as a possible trigger of insulin-dependent diabetes mellitus. *N Engl J Med* 1992;327:302-7.
6. Kolata G. How important is dietary calcium in preventing osteoporosis? *Science* 1986;233:519-20.
7. Zemel MB. Role of the sulfur-containing amino acids in protein-induced hypercalciuria in men. *J Nutr* 1981; 111:545.
8. Hegsted M, et al. Urinary calcium and calcium balance in young men as affected by level of protein and phosphorus intake. *J Nutr* 1981;111:553.
9. Mazess R. Bone mineral content of North Alaskan Eskimos. *Am J Clin Nutr* 1974;27:916-25.
10. Nielsen FH. Boron--an overlooked element of potential nutritional importnce. *Nutrition Today* Jan-Feb 1988;4-7.
11. Nielsen FH, Hunt CD, et al. Effect of dietary boron on mineral, estrogen, and testosterone metabolism in postmenopausal women. *FASEB J* 1987 1:394-97.
12. Simoons FJ. A geographic approach to senile cataracts: possible links with milk consumption, lactase activity, and galactose metabolism. *Digestive Diseases and Sciences* 1982;27(3):257-64.
13. Brenner BM, et al. Dietary protein intake and the progressive nature of kidney disease. *New Eng J Med* 1982;307(11):652:59.
14. Bosch JP, et al. Renal functional reserve in humans: effect of protein intake on glomerular filtration rate. *Am J Med* 1983;75:943-50.

15. Jones MG, et al. The effect of dietary protein on glomerular filtration rate in normal subjects. *Clin Nephrology* 1987;27(2):71-75.
16. Virag R, Bouilly P, Frydman D. Is impotence an arterial disorder? A study of arterial risk factors in 440 impotent men. *Lancet* 1985;1:181-84.

CHAPTER 7

1. Jaffe JH. Drug Addiction and Drug Abuse. In: Goodman LS, Gilman A. 1975. *The Pharmacological Basis of Therapeutics*. NY: Macmillan.
2. U.S. Department of Health and Human Services. 1987 *Sixth Special Report to the U.S. Congress on Alcohol and Health*. Washington, D.C.: US DHHS.
3. Chien, CP. Psychiatric treatment for geriatric patients: 'Pub' or drug? *Am J Psych* 1971;127:110.
4. von Wartburg JP, Buhler R. Alcoholism and Aldehydism. *New Biomedical Concepts* 1984;50(1):5-15.
5. Wurtman RJ. Aspartame: possible effect on seizure susceptibility. *Lancet* 1985;2:1060.
6. Camfield PR, Camfield CS, Dooley JM, Gordon K, Jollymore S, Weaver DF. Aspartame exacerbates EEG spike-wave discharge in children with generalized absence epilepsy: a double-blind controlled study. *Neurology* 1992; 42: 1000-03.
7. Janssen PJCM, van der Heijden CA. Aspartame: review of recent experimental and observational data. *Toxicology* 1988;50: 1-26
8. Yokogushi H, Wurtman RJ. Meal composition and plasma amino acid ratios: effect of various proteins on carbohydrates, and of various protein concentrations. *Metabolism* 1986;35(9):837-842.
9. Seltzer S, et al. The effects of dietary tryptophan on chronic maxillofacial pain and experimental pain tolerance. *J Psychiatric Res* 1983;17:181-86.
10. Seltzer S, et al. Alteration of human pain thresholds by nutritional manipulation and L-tryptophan supplementation. *Pain* 1982; 13:385-93.

CHAPTER 8

1. Walker A, Zimmerman MR, LEakey REF. A possible case of hyper-vitaminosis A in Homo erectus. *Nature* 1982;296(5854):248-50.

CHAPTER 9

1. Henderson MM, Kushi LH, Thompson DJ, et al. Feasibility of a randomized trial of a low-fat diet for the prevention of breast cancer: dietary compliance in the Women's Health Trial Vanguard Study. Prev Med 1990;19:115-33.
2. Willett WC, Hunter DJ, Stampfer MJ, et al. Dietary fat and fiber in relation to risk of breast cancer: an 8-year follow-up. JAMA 1992;268:2037-44.
3. The Alpha-tocopherol, beta-carotene cancer prevention study group. The effect of vitamin E and beta carotene on the incidence of lung cancer and other cancers in male smokers. N Engl J Med 1994;330:1029-35.

CHAPTER 10

1. Herbert V. Vitamin B-12; plant sources, requirements and assay. *Am J Clin Nutr* 1988;48:852-58.

CHAPTER 11

1. Schachter S. Recidivism and self-cure of smoking and obesity. *American Psychologist* 1982; 37 (4):436-44.
2. Kubler-Ross, Elisabeth. 1969. *On Death and Dying*. New York: MacMillan.

Index

Ask your store to carry these books,
or you may order directly from:

The Book Publishing Company   *Or call: 1-800-695-2241*
P.O. Box 99   *Please add $2.50 per book*
Summertown, TN 38483   *for shipping*

Almost-No Fat Cookbook	10.95
American Harvest	11.95
Burgers 'n Fries 'n Cinnamon Buns	6.95
Cookin' Healthy with One Foot Out the Door	8.95
Cooking with Gluten and Seitan	7.95
Ecological Cooking: Recipes to Save the Planet	10.95
Fabulous Beans	9.95
From A Traditional Greek Kitchen	9.95
Good Time Eatin' in Cajun Country	9.95
George Bernard Shaw Vegetarian Cookbook	8.95
Healthy Cook's Kitchen Companion	12.95
Holiday Diet Book	9.95
Instead of Chicken, Instead of Turkey:	9.95
Judy Brown's Guide to Natural Foods Cooking	10.95
Kids Can Cook	9.95
Murrieta Hot Springs Vegetarian Cookbook	9.95
New Farm Vegetarian Cookbook	8.95
Now & Zen Epicure	17.95
Olive Oil Cookery	11.95
Peaceful Cook	8.95
Physician's Slimming Guide, Neal D. Barnard, M..D	5.95
Also by Dr. Barnard:	
Foods That Cause You To Lose Weight	12.95
Live Longer, Live Better (90 min. cassette)	9.95
Beyond Animal Experiments (90 min. cassette)	9.95
Shiitake Way	7.95
Shoshoni Cookbook	12.95
Simply Heavenly	19.95
Soups For All Seasons	9.95
The Sprout Garden	8.95
Starting Over: Learning to Cook with Natural Foods	10.95
Tempeh Cookbook	10.95
Ten Talents (Vegetarian Cookbook)	18.95
Tofu Cookery	14.95
Tofu Quick & Easy	7.95
TVP® Cookbook	6.95
Uncheese Cookbook	11.95
Uprisings: The Whole Grain Bakers' Book	13.95
Vegetarian Cooking for People with Diabetes	10.95